Endoscopy in Inflammatory Bowel Disease

Editor

MARIA T. ABREU

GASTROINTESTINAL ENDOSCOPY CLINICS OF NORTH AMERICA

www.giendo.theclinics.com

Consulting Editor
CHARLES J. LIGHTDALE

October 2016 • Volume 26 • Number 4

ELSEVIER

1600 John F. Kennedy Boulevard • Suite 1800 • Philadelphia, Pennsylvania, 19103-2899

http://www.theclinics.com

GASTROINTESTINAL ENDOSCOPY CLINICS OF NORTH AMERICA Volume 26, Number 4
October 2016 ISSN 1052-5157, ISBN-13: 978-0-323-46310-2

Editor: Kerry Holland
Developmental Editor: Donald Mumford

Gastrointestinal Endoscopy Clinics of North America (ISSN 1052-5157) is published quarterly by Elsevier Inc., 360 Park Avenue South, New York, NY 10010-1710. Months of issue are January, April, July, and October. Business and Editorial Offices: 1600 John F. Kennedy Blvd., Suite 1800, Philadelphia, PA, 19103-2899. Periodicals postage paid at New York, NY and additional mailing offices. Subscription prices are $335.00 per year for US individuals, $538.00 per year for US institutions, $100.00 per year for US students and residents, $370.00 per year for Canadian individuals, $637.00 per year for Canadian institutions, $465.00 per year for international individuals, $637.00 per year for international institutions, and $245.00 per year for Canadian and foreign students/residents. To receive student/resident rate, orders must be accompanied by name of affiliated institution, date of term, and the *signature* of program/residency coordinator on institution letterhead. Orders will be billed at individual rate until proof of status is received. Foreign air speed delivery is included in all *Clinics* subscription prices. All prices are subject to change without notice. **POSTMASTER:** Send address change to *Gastrointestinal Endoscopy Clinics of North America*, Elsevier Health Sciences Division, Subscription Customer Service, 3251 Riverport Lane, Maryland Heights, MO 63043. **Customer Service: 1-800-654-2452 (US). From outside the United States, call 1-314-447-8871. Fax: 1-314-447-8029. E-mail: JournalsCustomerService-usa@elsevier.com (for print support) or JournalsOnlineSupport-usa@elsevier.com (for online support).**

Reprints. For copies of 100 or more, of articles in this publication, please contact the Commercial Reprints Department, Elsevier Inc., 360 Park Avenue South, New York, NY 10010-1710. Tel. 212-633-3874; Fax: 212-633-3820; E-mail: reprints@elsevier.com.

Gastrointestinal Endoscopy Clinics of North America is covered in *Excerpta Medica, MEDLINE/PubMed (Index Medicus), and MEDLINE/MEDLARS.*

Contributors

CONSULTING EDITOR

CHARLES J. LIGHTDALE, MD
Professor of Medicine, Division of Digestive and Liver Diseases, Columbia University Medical Center, New York, New York

EDITOR

MARIA T. ABREU, MD
Director, Crohn's and Colitis Center; Professor of Medicine; Professor of Microbiology and Immunology, University of Miami Miller School of Medicine, Miami, Florida

AUTHORS

SHERINE M. ABDALLA, MD
Resident, Department of Medicine, Jackson Memorial Hospital, University of Miami, Miami, Florida

BELÉN BELTRÁN, MD, PhD
Gastroenterology Department, Department of Digestive Disease, Centro de Investigación Biomédica en Red de Enfermedades Hepáticas y Digestivas (CIBERehd), La Fe University and Polytechnic Hospital, Valencia, Spain

DAVID G. BINION, MD, AGAF, FACG
Professor of Medicine, Clinical and Translational Science; Co-Director of IBD Center; Director of Translational IBD Research; Director of Nutrition Support Service, Division of Gastroenterology, Hepatology and Nutrition, UPMC-Presbyterian Hospital, University of Pittsburgh School of Medicine, Pittsburgh, Pennsylvania

ANNA M. BUCHNER, MD, PhD
Assistant Professor of Medicine, Division of Gastroenterology, University of Pennsylvania, Philadelphia, Pennsylvania

DAN CARTER, MD
Department of Gastroenterology, Sheba Medical Center, Tel Hashomer, Israel; Sackler School of Medicine, Tel Aviv University, Tel Aviv, Israel

ROBIN L. DALAL, MD
Gastroenterology Fellow, Division of Gastroenterology, Vanderbilt University Medical Center, Nashville, Tennessee

MARLA C. DUBINSKY, MD
Professor of Pediatrics, Division of Pediatric Gastroenterology and Hepatology, Susan and Leonard Feinstein IBD Clinical Center, Icahn School of Medicine at Mount Sinai, New York, New York

ABRAHAM RAMI ELIAKIM, MD
Department of Gastroenterology, Sheba Medical Center, Tel Hashomer, Israel; Sackler School of Medicine, Tel Aviv University, Tel Aviv, Israel

REBECCA A. FAUSEL, MD
The Dr. Henry D. Janowitz Division of Gastroenterology, Icahn School of Medicine at Mount Sinai, New York, New York

JANA G. HASHASH, MD, MSc
Assistant Professor of Medicine, Division of Gastroenterology, Hepatology and Nutrition, UPMC-Presbyterian Hospital, University of Pittsburgh School of Medicine, Pittsburgh, Pennsylvania

MARISA IBORRA, MD, PhD
Gastroenterology Department, Department of Digestive Disease, Centro de Investigación Biomédica en Red de Enfermedades Hepáticas y Digestivas (CIBERehd), La Fe University and Polytechnic Hospital, Valencia, Spain

GORAV KALRA, MD
Gastroenterology Fellow, Department of Medicine, Jackson Memorial Hospital, University of Miami, Miami, Florida

DAVID H. KERMAN, MD
Assistant Professor of Clinical Medicine; Director, Gastroenterology Fellowship Program, Division of Gastroenterology, University of Miami Miller School of Medicine, Miami, Florida

URI KOPYLOV, MD
Department of Gastroenterology, Sheba Medical Center, Tel Hashomer, Israel; Sackler School of Medicine, Tel Aviv University, Tel Aviv, Israel

ASHER KORNBLUTH, MD
Clinical Professor of Medicine, The Dr. Henry D. Janowitz Division of Gastroenterology, Icahn School of Medicine at Mount Sinai, New York, New York

JOHN A. MARTIN, MD, FASGE
Associate Professor; Associate Chair for Endoscopy; Senior Associate Consultant, Division of Gastroenterology and Hepatology, Mayo Clinic, Rochester, Minnesota

BAHA MOSHIREE, MD, MS-CI
Associate Professor of Medicine, Department of Medicine, University of Miami Miller School of Medicine, Miami, Florida

ALAN C. MOSS, MD, FACG, FEBG, AGAF, FRCPI
Associate Professor of Medicine, Harvard Medical School, Boston, Massachusetts

PILAR NOS, MD, PhD
Gastroenterology Department, Department of Digestive Disease, Centro de Investigación Biomédica en Red de Enfermedades Hepáticas y Digestivas (CIBERehd), La Fe University and Polytechnic Hospital, Valencia, Spain

ROBERT D. ODZE, MD, FRCPC
Chief, Gastrointestinal Pathology; Professor of Pathology, Brigham and Women's Hospital, Harvard Medical School, Boston, Massachusetts

DEEPA T. PATIL, MD
Associate Professor of Pathology, Cleveland Clinic, Cleveland, Ohio

NAYANTARA COELHO-PRABHU, MBBS
Assistant Professor, Division of Gastroenterology and Hepatology, Mayo Clinic, Rochester, Minnesota

DAVID A. SCHWARTZ, MD
Director IBD Center, Professor of Medicine; Division of Gastroenterology, Vanderbilt University Medical Center, Nashville, Tennessee

BO SHEN, MD
The Ed and Joey Story Endowed Chair and Professor of Medicine, The Interventional IBD (i-IBD) Unit, Digestive Disease and Surgery Institute, The Cleveland Clinic Foundation, Cleveland, Ohio

MICHAEL B. WALLACE, MD, MPH
Professor of Medicine, Division of Gastroenterology and Hepatology, Mayo Clinic, Jacksonville, Florida

Contents

of the timing and purpose of endoscopic evaluation in postoperative CD patients and pragmatic information regarding interpretation of endoscopic findings at the different types of surgical anastomoses after ileocecal resection.

Perianal fistula occurs frequently in the Crohn's disease population. Therapy for fistulas has changed through the years from primarily surgical management to multidisciplinary management among gastroenterologists, radiologists, and surgeons. Gastroenterologists play a role in assisting with diagnosis through endoscopic ultrasound and assessment of luminal disease activity, providing medical therapy including biologic therapy and antibiotics, and coordinating the multidisciplinary care with surgical and radiologic colleagues.

The intestinal microbiome plays an important role in the pathogenesis of inflammatory bowel disease (IBD). We are able to use the microbiome as a therapeutic target with use of fecal microbiota transplantation (FMT) for cure of recurrent *Clostridium difficile* infection. Given our ability to target the dysbiotic state with FMT, its use as therapy in IBD has tremendous potential. This overview discusses the practical considerations of FMT therapy with respect to our current understanding of safety and efficacy in IBD, screening for donors and recipients, specimen handling and storage, methods of delivery, and regulatory considerations.

Patients with inflammatory bowel disease (IBD) suffer frequently from functional bowel diseases (FBD) and motility disorders. Management of FBD and motility disorders in IBD combined with continued treatment of a patient's IBD symptoms will likely lead to better clinical outcomes and improve the patient's quality of life. The goals of this review are to summarize the most recent literature on motility disturbances in patients with IBD and to give a brief overview of the ranges of motility disturbances, from reflux disease to anorectal disorders, and discuss their diagnosis and specific management.

Stricture formation occurs in up to 40% of patients with inflammatory bowel disease (IBD). Patients are often symptomatic, resulting in significant morbidity, hospitalizations, and loss of productivity. Strictures can be managed endoscopically in addition to traditional surgical management (sphincteroplasty or resection of the affected bowel segments). About 3%

to 5% patients with IBD develop primary sclerosing cholangitis (PSC), which results in stricture formation in the biliary tree, managed for the most part by endoscopic therapies. In this article, we discuss endoscopic management of strictures both in the alimentary tract and biliary tree in patients with IBD and/or PSC.

GASTROINTESTINAL ENDOSCOPY CLINICS OF NORTH AMERICA

THE CLINICS ARE AVAILABLE ONLINE!
Access your subscription at:
www.theclinics.com

Foreword

The Key Roles of Endoscopy in Inflammatory Bowel Disease

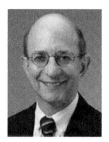

Charles J. Lightdale, MD
Consulting Editor

New scientific insights into the pathogenesis of inflammation and autoimmune diseases, including inflammatory bowel disease, have led to a new era in the management of Crohn disease and ulcerative colitis. These discoveries have enabled better application of older anti-inflammatory agents and immunomodulators, and of course, have resulted in the introduction of novel biological agents, starting with infliximab, the monoclonal antibody to tumor necrosis factor-α. Multiple biological agents are now available to gastroenterologists treating inflammatory bowel disease, and many more are in the pharmaceutical development pipeline. At the same time, there is increasing evidence of the effects of the gut microbiome on the bowel mucosa in inflammatory bowel disease, and new treatments have emerged in an effort to modify the bacterial environment.

Remarkably, the roles of endoscopy have actually increased in this new era in management of Crohn disease and ulcerative colitis. At the same time, the demands on the endoscopist have significantly expanded for more careful systematic inspection and classification, and for proper application of advanced imaging, endoscopic biopsy, resection, and stricture dilation. It seemed clear to me that a new issue of the *Gastrointestinal Endoscopy Clinics of North America* on the subject of "Endoscopy in Inflammatory Bowel Disease" was needed. Dr Maria Abreu, an astute and thoughtful clinician and researcher, and a valued and prominent leader in the field, is the guest editor for this issue. She has chosen a truly comprehensive list of topics covering the multiple ways that endoscopy can assist in management of patients with inflammatory bowel disease and has gathered an extraordinary group of expert authors. There is much to be learned, and I strongly urge gastroenterologists and colorectal surgeons to read this issue in its entirety. This is critical reading for you and will ensure that you

Gastrointest Endoscopy Clin N Am 26 (2016) xiii–xiv
http://dx.doi.org/10.1016/j.giec.2016.07.002
1052-5157/16/© 2016 Published by Elsevier Inc.

giendo.theclinics.com

are up-to-date in applying endoscopy correctly for the benefit of your patients in the current time and into the future.

Charles J. Lightdale, MD
Department of Medicine
Columbia University Medical Center
161 Fort Washington Avenue
New York, NY 10032, USA

E-mail address:
CJL18@columbia.edu

Preface

Endoscopy in Inflammatory Bowel Disease

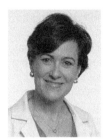

Maria T. Abreu, MD
Editor

As a gastroenterologist who specializes in inflammatory bowel disease (IBD), I call myself a "boutique" endoscopist. I primarily do endoscopies on patients with IBD and have come to realize, especially through the eyes of our fellows, how complicated it can be. Unlike a normal screening colonoscopy, gastroenterologists must take into account that most patients with IBD will take a lot longer for an endoscopy, and there is often a lot of work to be done. The work can take the form of many biopsies, chromoendoscopy, or dilations of strictures. I always explain to my fellows that endoscopy is an extension of the physical examination and that you need to have a plan for what you are looking for and what you intend to do about it.

The first article in this issue deals with a patient's very first endoscopy. Gastroenterologists who are performing an endoscopy on a patient with diarrhea or other gastrointestinal symptoms consistent with IBD must have a plan for what they intend to biopsy and what stool studies to send off. During that first endoscopy, it is critical to get into the terminal ileum and to biopsy both normal and abnormal mucosa throughout the colon. I most often use a pediatric colonoscope for all of my procedures simply because it makes it easier to get into a terminal ileum, especially if it is inflamed. If it is a patient I have scoped previously, I will make a note to myself in the endoscopy report if I think an adult colonoscope is better for that patient.

In a patient with ulcerative colitis, especially longstanding ulcerative colitis, biopsies become essential as well as a very careful look at the mucosa in search of mucosal changes of dysplasia. We have included thoughtful articles in this issue on the use of modern technologies, such as confocal laser endomicroscopy, which will allow us to identify very small foci of abnormalities or to map out the limits of an abnormal area once identified. I would argue that even high-definition white-light endoscopy is very superior to our old technology for identifying abnormal mucosa. It is better to be safe than sorry and to biopsy areas that look abnormal. A recent study found that fecal biotherapy was effective in the treatment of ulcerative colitis. We

Gastrointest Endoscopy Clin N Am 26 (2016) xv–xvi
http://dx.doi.org/10.1016/j.giec.2016.07.001
1052-5157/16/© 2016 Published by Elsevier Inc.

have dedicated one article on the data for fecal biotherapy in ulcerative colitis with and without *Clostridium difficile* infection with a focus on "how to" perform these procedures.

In Crohn's disease, most of the endoscopy revolves around identifying where the patient has disease and the severity of that disease. There are validated endoscopy-reporting tools that allow us to grade the endoscopy and are easily accessible to most gastroenterologists, especially since some of the most commonly used endoscopy reporting software have the endoscopy indices embedded in the program with pull-down menus to fill in the data. This becomes very important to track the patients over time and to have an objective way to compare what their endoscopy has shown previously. It also allows one to communicate with other doctors regarding the severity of the patient's disease.

In postoperative Crohn's disease, we are trying to identify inflammation in the neoterminal ileum and occasionally at the anastomosis itself. In this issue, you will find a very detailed article on the different types of anastomoses that occur in Crohn's disease, but, in general, except for an end-to-end anastomosis, which is rarely done these days, the gastroenterologist is going to have to spend time to identify the neoterminal ileum. Often it is at a very sharp angle to the remainder of the colon, requiring the gastroenterologist to literally make a U turn to get into the neoterminal ileum. Without that information, the colonoscopy is of no value. Commonly, patients with Crohn's disease who have had surgery will have a stricture at the ileocolic anastomosis, whether it is from ischemia during healing or from recurrence of the disease. We now commonly dilate these strictures, especially when they are not inflamed, using through-the-scope balloons. Dilation can delay the need or prevent the need for another surgery if the disease is limited to the anastomosis.

One of the most common reasons that we are performing endoscopy in patients with IBD is to assess for mucosal healing. Almost by definition, this means having an accurate description and preferably numerical score for how severe the inflammation was before the intervention so that one has a point of comparison afterwards. We have authors that have dealt in this issue with mucosal healing and how to interpret it and the improvement in outcomes in patients who achieve mucosal healing. Like everything in life, there has to be a balance of achieving the greatest degree of mucosal improvement while using medications that are safe and well tolerated for a particular patient. In addition to endoscopy, we cover noninvasive ways to monitor intestinal inflammation through the use of biochemical markers and fecal markers, which have become much more common these days and which can serve to diminish the need for such frequent endoscopy. Patients may also experience many symptoms even when they are in remission. We have provided a fascinating article on motility and functional disorders that arise in IBD patients and need separate management.

I hope that all of you will take some pearls from the accompanying articles. I believe that they will improve your endoscopic strategies for these challenging patients with IBD.

Maria T. Abreu, MD
Crohn's and Colitis Center
University of Miami Miller School of Medicine
Miami, FL 33136, USA

E-mail address:
mabreu1@med.miami.edu

The First Endoscopy in Suspected Inflammatory Bowel Disease

Rebecca A. Fausel, MD[a,*], Asher Kornbluth, MD[b],
Marla C. Dubinsky, MD[c]

KEYWORDS

- Endoscopy • Colonoscopy • Inflammatory bowel disease • Crohn's disease
- Ulcerative colitis • Backwash ileitis • Ileoscopy

KEY POINTS

- The initial colonoscopy in IBD should include a careful perianal inspection and digital rectal examination, to assess for findings associated with perianal Crohn's disease.
- It is important to perform a thorough and systematic assessment of the mucosa throughout the colon and ileum to accurately assess the pattern and extent of disease.
- The use of a validated endoscopic scoring system for grading of endoscopic IBD activity is important for improved standardization and communication of endoscopy findings, for monitoring endoscopic response to therapy, and for prognosis.
- Histologic evaluation should include assessment for features of chronicity, including crypt architectural distortion, basal plasmacytosis, and increased cellularity of the lamina propria, and can be essential in distinguishing IBD from acute self-limited colitis.
- Upper endoscopy with biopsies should be performed in all pediatric patients with suspected IBD, and in adult patients with suspected IBD and upper gastrointestinal symptoms.

Conflict of Interest/Disclosure: Dr M.C. Dubinsky is a consultant for Janssen, AbbVie, UCB, Takeda, Celgene, Genentech, Boehringer Ingelheim, and Prometheus Laboratories. Dr A. Kornbluth has no relevant conflicts of interest or financial disclosures.
[a] The Dr. Henry D. Janowitz Division of Gastroenterology, Icahn School of Medicine at Mount Sinai, One Gustave L. Levy Place, Box 1069, New York, NY 10029-6574, USA; [b] The Dr. Henry D. Janowitz Division of Gastroenterology, Icahn School of Medicine at Mount Sinai, 1150 Fifth Avenue, Suite 1B, New York, NY 10128, USA; [c] Division of Pediatric Gastroenterology and Hepatology, Susan and Leonard Feinstein IBD Clinical Center, Icahn School of Medicine at Mount Sinai, 17 East 102nd Street, 5th Floor, New York, NY 10029, USA
* Corresponding author.
E-mail address: rebecca.fausel@mountsinai.org

INTRODUCTION

The diagnosis of inflammatory bowel disease (IBD) is based on established clinical, endoscopic, radiologic, and histologic features. In a patient presenting with suspected IBD, the initial endoscopic evaluation is an indispensable tool, valuable in determining the correct disease diagnosis, extent and severity of disease, and prognosis. The distinction between Crohn's disease (CD) and ulcerative colitis (UC) is made accurately in greater than 85% of patients, and this distinction can have important ramifications for future medical and surgical therapies.[1] The American Society for Gastrointestinal Endoscopy guidelines recommend a full colonoscopy with ileal intubation in all patients with a clinical presentation suggestive of IBD, unless contraindicated by the presence of severe colitis or toxic megacolon.[2,3] This article discusses important macroscopic findings on the first endoscopy in suspected IBD, histopathologic interpretation of biopsy specimens, endoscopic scoring systems, and prognostic implications.

PERIANAL EXAMINATION

Patients with IBD can present with a myriad of symptoms including diarrhea, rectal bleeding, abdominal pain, nausea, vomiting, weight loss, and fecal urgency. Colonoscopic evaluation is one of the first steps in assessment of these symptoms. Before the initial colonoscopy, it is important to perform a careful perianal inspection and digital rectal examination because it may reveal clues to the diagnosis of CD, including the following[4]:

- Anal skin tags, particularly type 1
- Anal fissure
- Deep anal canal ulcer
- Perianal fistula
- Perianal abscess
- Anorectal stricture

Type 1 anal skin tags are sometimes referred to as "elephant ears" and can have a varied appearance. They are present in up to 40% of patients with IBD, occurring in patients with CD, but rarely in UC.[5] They are often painless but can become painful, at times associated with exacerbation of colonic disease.[6]

Anal fissures, ulcerations in the lining of the anal canal distal to the dentate line, are present in about 30% of patients with perianal disease.[7] As with idiopathic anal fissures, these most often occur in the midline but can also occur eccentrically. Multiple, nonhealing, painless, or eccentrically located anal fissures should raise the suspicion for a diagnosis of CD.[8]

A hallmark of perianal involvement in CD is perianal fistulae, which occur in up to 45% to 50% of patients over the course of their disease and may be a presenting symptom in 20% to 30% of patients. It is more common in patients with Crohn's colitis.[9] Fistulae can arise from inflamed or infected anal glands or from penetration of fissures or ulcers of the rectum or anal canal. They may appear as abnormal perianal openings or as small pustules. Gentle compression adjacent to the orifice may express purulent material or stool. It is important to look for areas of fluctuance and tenderness, or pain on digital rectal examination, which could indicate the presence of an abscess. The development of a new perianal rigid mass in a patient with longstanding perianal disease should raise the suspicion of a perianal squamous cell carcinoma.

EXAMINATION OF COLONIC MUCOSA DURING ENDOSCOPY

The normal colon lining appears smooth and glistening salmon-pink in color, with a transparent surface mucosa and a visible network of branching vessels beneath (**Fig. 1**).[1] Assessment of the mucosa should include an assessment of the vascular pattern, and evaluation for the presence of erythema, edema, granularity, friability, ulcerations, and spontaneous bleeding. In IBD and other types of intestinal inflammation, the normal vascular pattern can be obliterated and the mucosa can develop the aforementioned characteristics of inflammation, even deep crater-like ulcerations in severe cases. The macroscopic appearance on endoscopy is not conclusive for the diagnosis of IBD, but in conjunction with histology and clinical presentation, it may provide important information in considering a broad differential diagnosis that includes infectious enterocolitis, ischemia,[1,10,11] drug-induced injury,[12] Behçet disease,[10,11] and segmental colitis associated with diverticulosis (**Table 1**).[13,14]

The earliest response to tissue injury in UC is an increase in surface blood flow leading to erythema, vascular congestion, and edema, which can appear as "wet sandpaper."[1] On the first colonoscopy, the typical endoscopic feature is the presence of continuous inflammation extending proximally from the anal verge, often characterized by erythema, edema, and ulceration (**Fig. 2**). The degree of inflammation classically increases in a proximal to distal pattern. There is often a line of demarcation at the proximal extent of disease, with an abrupt transition to normal mucosa.[3]

The earliest endoscopically visible lesion in CD consists of very small punched-out ulcers in an otherwise normal-appearing mucosa, also called aphthous ulcerations. As disease severity increases, deeper ulcers involving all or part of the colonic wall can develop. Cobblestoning is a hallmark feature of CD that occurs when long linear or serpiginous ulcers course along the longitudinal axis of the colon, with intervening areas of normal or inflamed tissue (**Fig. 3**). Lesions in CD are often discontinuous and adjacent to normal tissue, resulting in "skip lesions."

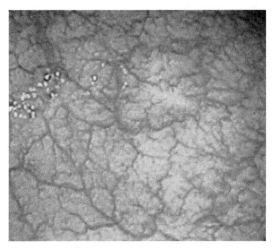

Fig. 1. Endoscopic appearance of normal colonic mucosa.

Table 1
Selected differential diagnosis of ileocolonic inflammation

Differential Diagnosis	Classic Clinical Presentation	Endoscopy Findings	Histology Findings
Cytomegalovirus colitis	• Acute/subacute bloody or nonbloody diarrhea • Fever and abdominal pain • Almost always in immunosuppressed	• Patchy erythema • Discrete punched out, well-demarcated ulcerations of varying size and depth	• Cytomegalic inclusion bodies (biopsy from edges) • Immunohistochemistry
Clostridium difficile colitis	• Acute/subacute nonbloody diarrhea • Often associated with recent antibiotic use • Can be community acquired without antibiotic use	• Yellow membrane overlying mucosal surface • Small elevated cream/yellow colored plaques • Nonulcerated mucosa between plaques	• Polymorphonuclear exudate with "volcano" lesions
Other infectious colitides (ie, *Campylobacter*, *Salmonella*, *Shigella*, *Escherichia coli*, *Entamoeba histolytica*, sexually transmitted proctitides, intestinal tuberculosis)	• Bloody or nonbloody diarrhea • Fevers and abdominal pain • Self-limited illness <4 wk (exceptions: tuberculosis, *Campylobacter*, schistosomiasis, amebiasis) • Recent travel or other exposures	• Often indistinguishable from IBD • May have yellowish exudate or free purulent material • Intensely reddened surface mucosa • Patchy inflammation within same segment; may see aphthae	• Can be indistinguishable from early IBD • Intense neutrophilic infiltrate • Focal cryptitis • Absence of basal plasmacytosis • Absence of crypt architectural changes
Ischemic colitis	• Acute onset of cramping abdominal pain, diarrhea, and hematochezia • Elderly patients • Peripheral vascular disease, hematologic or cardiologic impairment, recent vascular surgery	• Affects "watershed areas" -> most common in descending colon near splenic flexure; can occur in sigmoid and right colon • Mild: edema, loss of vascular pattern, may see aphthae • Severe: plum-red to blue-black discoloration, even necrosis and gangrene	• Variable inflammatory component • Hemosiderin-laden macrophages • Hemorrhage into mucosa • Preferential damage to surface epithelium • In severe: mucosal necrosis with sloughing

Nonsteroidal anti-inflammatory drug-induced injury	• May present with abdominal pain, hematochezia • Often no GI symptoms • Medication history	• Discrete ulcerations surrounded by normal mucosa • Can involve any segment of GI tract	• Primary mucosal ulceration • Mild villous blunting or superficial erosion • No associated vascular damage or transmural inflammation • Prominent apoptosis and increased intraepithelial lymphocyte counts, sometimes with predominant eosinophils
Behçet disease	• GI symptoms similar to IBD • Oral and genital ulcers • May have multisystem involvement caused by vasculitis	• Appearance similar to CD with discrete ulcerations	• Punched out or flask-shaped ulcers that can involve submucosa and muscular propria • Normal adjacent tissue • Vasculitis may be seen adjacent to ulceration
Segmental colitis associated with diverticulosis	• Lower left quadrant cramping pain, hematochezia, diarrhea • May be asymptomatic • Older patients • More common in men	• Inflammation of interdiverticular mucosa, usually in sigmoid • Rectal sparing • Varied endoscopic appearance and severity • Edema, erythema, loss of normal vascular pattern in some cases • Aphthous ulcerations or diffuse ulceration in other cases	• Chronic inflammatory changes • Varied histologic appearance depending on endoscopic pattern • Basal plasmacytosis, mixed inflammation in lamina propria, crypt architectural distortion, crypt abscesses • Can have epithelioid granulomas and lymphohistiocytic vasculitis

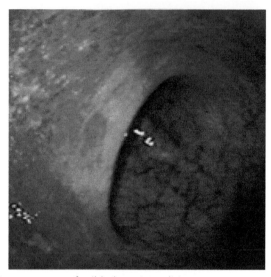

Fig. 2. Endoscopic appearance of mild ulcerative colitis.

The index colonoscopy and biopsies are accurate in distinguishing CD from UC in 89% of cases.[15] However, this differentiation is challenging at times. Features that raise suspicion of CD include the following:

- Rectal sparing
- Patchy colitis or skip lesions
- Discrete ileal ulcerations
- Isolated ileal inflammation
- Extensive ileal involvement

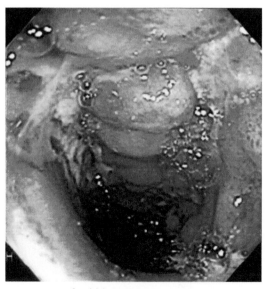

Fig. 3. Endoscopic appearance of cobblestoning.

- Ileal or ileocecal (IC) valve narrowing
- Cobblestoning of mucosa
- Long linear or serpiginous ulcers
- Deep ulcers
- Aphthous ulcers

Many of these features are suggestive, but not confirmatory, for a diagnosis of CD. For example, cobblestoning and deep ulcers can be seen in severe UC.

In approximately 10% of patients, their colonic disease cannot be classified into either of these categories, and it is termed IBD, type unclassified. The distinguishing endoscopic findings are particularly useful at the time of diagnosis, because the endoscopic appearance can change with treatment and patchy healing can occur. In one study of patients with UC, 44% had patchy colitis and 13% had rectal sparing after treatment.[16]

CECAL PATCH

Despite the general tenet that patchy or segmental colitis is consistent with CD, isolated inflammatory changes around the appendiceal orifice without adjacent colonic inflammation are seen in UC. This finding is termed a cecal patch or a periappendiceal red patch. The rate of cecal patch ranges from 8%[17] to 75%[18] in some studies. It tends to parallel the inflammatory activity seen in the distal colon.[19] It is more commonly seen in younger patients with longer disease duration, and thus far has not been shown to have any impact on disease remission, relapse, proximal extension, or dysplasia or cancer risk.[20,21]

RECTAL SPARING

Rectal sparing is classically thought to be consistent with CD. However, atypical endoscopic findings at diagnosis can occur in a subset of patients with UC, more commonly in the pediatric population.[22-24] Although histologic sparing is less common, macroscopic and histologic sparing have been reported. In children, relative rectal sparing (defined as reduced histologic severity and chronicity compared with more proximal colon) occurs in up to 23%, whereas full macroscopic rectal sparing occurs in 5% or less.[22-24] In addition, patchy inflammation throughout the colon may occur in pediatric patients with UC before therapy.[23]

In adults, this phenomenon is less frequently recognized, although more than half of patients with primary sclerosing cholangitis with UC have rectal sparing, possibly representing a separate disease phenotype.[25] In a 2014 Korean study, 19.2% of patients with UC had patchy inflammation based on macroscopic visualization alone on the initial colonoscopy, with 3.3% rectal sparing.[26] Another study showed rectal sparing at diagnosis to be rare in adults.[27] In general, the presence of rectal sparing at first colonoscopy should suggest a diagnosis of CD.[3]

INTESTINAL STRICTURE

Although most patients present with pure inflammatory disease at diagnosis, 11% of patients with CD have strictures at initial evaluation.[28] Strictures are most commonly located in the ileum and ileocecal valve; however, they can occur at any site in the gastrointestinal (GI) tract. Per the National Cooperative Crohn's Disease Study, small bowel strictures occur in 25% of patients and colonic strictures in 10% of patients, although these numbers preceded the use of immunosuppressive and biologic drug treatment.[28]

When a stricture is encountered in CD, it is important to assess for inflammation of the stricture itself and the adjacent mucosa. If traversable, the length and diameter of the stricture should be estimated. Multiple biopsies should be taken within and around the stricture to assess for dysplasia, with special attention paid to colonic strictures. Stricturing and penetrating disease complications may occur in the same patient, but fistulas can be difficult to visualize on colonoscopy.[29]

Colonic strictures can also occur in patients with UC, but they are far less common, estimated in about 1% of patients (**Fig. 4**). The historical teaching is that these strictures should be considered malignant until proven otherwise. A retrospective study of 1156 patients with UC showed a 24% prevalence of malignancy within UC strictures.[30] A more recent case control study showed a much lower rate of malignancy, but the rate was elevated compared with patients without strictures.[31] If encountered on the first colonoscopy, it is imperative to carefully survey all UC strictures with multiple biopsies.

Inability to traverse a stricture with a standard adult colonoscope should prompt downsizing to the smallest caliber scope available.[32] Balloon stricture dilation can be carried out to allow passage through a stricture but carries a risk of perforation especially if the stricture and the surrounding mucosa are ulcerated. A recent systematic review and meta-analysis showed a 4% risk of major adverse events.[33]

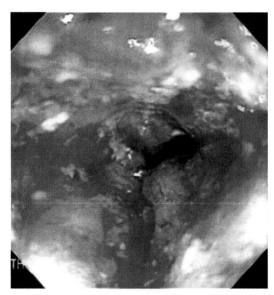

Fig. 4. Endoscopic appearance of ulcerated stricture in ulcerative colitis.

ILEOSCOPY

Ileoscopy is a valuable tool to assess for ileal inflammation and to distinguish ileal CD from backwash ileitis.[2,3] In patients presenting with diarrhea, the yield of ileoscopy ranges from 5% to 48%.[34] In one study, endoscopic lesions of the terminal ileum were found in 48%, more than one-third of which had no colonic involvement, underlining the importance of ileal intubation for correct diagnosis.[35] The maneuver adds an average of 3.4 minutes to the procedure time and adds minimal risk.[34] However, ileoscopy may be falsely negative if a patient's small bowel disease does not involve the most distal portion of the ileum, and alternative evaluation with MRI enterography or capsule endoscopy may be required.[35] There is currently no evidence to determine whether the choice of instrument (adult versus pediatric colonoscope) impacts the success of ileal intubation when Crohn's disease is suspected.

Inflammation of the terminal ileum is suggestive of CD, although 17% of patients with UC can develop a "backwash ileitis."[36] The term evolved from the belief that this inflammation results from exposure to cecal contents, although its true pathogenesis remains poorly understood.

There are features on macroscopic and histologic examination of the ileum that assist in distinguishing backwash ileitis from CD (**Table 2**).[36] There has been report of a possible association of backwash ileitis with aggressive disease course and primary sclerosing cholangitis.[37] One study reported an increased rate of dysplasia and carcinoma, but this has not been confirmed in other reports.[36,38] The presence of backwash ileitis does not seem to affect pouch outcome in patients with UC who undergo restorative proctocolectomy.[39]

Table 2
Features of backwash ileitis versus Crohn's ileitis

Typical Features	Backwash Ileitis	Crohn's Disease
Macroscopic	• Mild erythema and edema • Short contiguous segment • Rare superficial erosions • Most often in setting of moderate-severe pancolitis	• Discrete or aphthous ulcerations • Extensive or patchy ulceration • Severity may be greater than cecal inflammation • Strictures of ileocecal valve or terminal ileum
Histopathologic	• Generally mild • Mixed inflammatory infiltrate of lamina propria • Villous atrophy may occur • Scattered crypt abscesses • No crypt distortion	• Lymphoplasmacytic inflammation in lamina propria • Granulomas (not always present) • Architectural distortion • Submucosal inflammation • Fissuring ulceration • Pyloric metaplasia

CLASSIFICATION SYSTEMS AND ENDOSCOPIC SCORING IN INFLAMMATORY BOWEL DISEASE

An accurate and thorough description of endoscopic findings is critical for guiding therapeutic decision making and monitoring response to treatment. Devlin and colleagues[40] recently published a comprehensive list of recommended elements for quality IBD colonoscopy reporting based on consensus from a panel of expert IBD gastroenterologists.

Classification systems also help to standardize the interpretation of endoscopic findings. The Montreal Classification describes the distribution of disease in UC and CD with excellent interobserver agreement.[41,42] For UC, the classification includes E1, proctitis; E2, left-sided UC distal to splenic flexure; and E3, extensive UC extending proximal to splenic flexure. At diagnosis, approximately 30% to 50% of patients have disease limited to the rectum or sigmoid colon, 20% to 30% have left-sided colitis, and 20% have pancolitis.[43]

CD can involve any segment of the GI tract from the mouth to the anus. Approximately 80% of patients have small bowel involvement, usually in the distal ileum. One-third of patients have ileitis exclusively, 50% of patients have ileocolitis, and 20% have disease limited to the colon.[9,43,44] The disease location tends to be stable over time.[9] The

Montreal Classification for CD includes age at diagnosis, localization of disease, and disease behavior.[41] The classification for disease location includes the following:

- L1: Terminal ileum (disease limited to terminal ileum with or without spillover into cecum)
- L2: Colon
- L3: Ileocolonic
- L4: Upper GI tract (can be added to L1–L3)
- Additional indicator of perianal disease (p)

In addition to documenting disease distribution, it is important to assess the endoscopic disease activity. Endoscopic scoring systems seek to reduce the variability of this assessment. In UC, the Mayo score combines an endoscopic scale with clinical categories including stool frequency, rectal bleeding, and physician global assessment. It is commonly used in clinical trials, but interobserver agreement among expert IBD gastroenterologists is suboptimal.[45] The endoscopic subscore is a scale from 0 to 3, based on the most severe segment of inflammation.

- Mayo Score 0: Normal mucosa or inactive colitis
- Mayo Score 1: Mild friability, reduction in normal vascular pattern, erythema
- Mayo Score 2: Significant erythema, friability, erosions, complete loss of vascular pattern
- Mayo Score 3: Frank ulceration and/or spontaneous bleeding

The Modified Mayo Clinic Endoscopic Score has been developed to account for disease distribution. The colon is divided into five segments. The endoscopic subscore for each segment is added together, multiplied by the maximal extent of examination (maximum of five if entire colon examined), then divided by the number of segments with active inflammation. The Modified Mayo Clinic Endoscopic Score has not yet been validated, but does correlate with clinical, biologic, and histologic activity.[46,47]

Another validated tool, with good interobserver and intraobserver reliability, is the Ulcerative Colitis Endoscopy Index of Severity (UCEIS) (**Table 3**).[48] This scoring system is responsive to clinical change, and can help predict clinical outcome in acute severe colitis.[49] Either the Mayo score or UCEIS can be used for grading the disease activity seen on index colonoscopy; however, the UCEIS may have less interobserver variation and may be more responsive to change.[49]

Table 3
Ulcerative colitis endoscopic index of severity

Variable	Score 0	Score 1	Score 2	Score 3
Vascular pattern	Normal	Patchy obliteration	Complete obliteration	N/A
Bleeding	None	Mucosal	Luminal: mild	Luminal: moderate to severe
Erosions and ulcers	None	Erosions ≤5 mm	Superficial ulcer >5 mm	Deep excavated defect/ulcer

Most severe lesions are scored.
Scores are added for final sum.
Data from Travis SP, Schnell D, Krzeski P, et al. Developing an instrument to assess the endoscopic severity of ulcerative colitis: the Ulcerative Colitis Endoscopy Index of Severity (UCEIS). Gut 2012;61(4):535–42.

In CD, there are two validated endoscopic scoring systems, the Crohn's Disease Endoscopic Index of Severity and the Simple Endoscopic Score for Crohn's Disease (SES-CD). The Crohn's Disease Endoscopic Index of Severity includes categories of deep ulcerations, superficial ulcerations, length of ulcerated mucosa, and length of diseased mucosa. Its use is limited by significant complexity and need for specialized training.[50,51] The Simple Endoscopic Score for Crohn's Disease is a simplified version (**Table 4**), but still involves scoring multiple segments and multiple variables.[52] Both scoring systems have excellent intraobserver and interobserver reliability, although their responsiveness to therapy has not been established.[53] The use of these scoring systems is important for classifying the initial disease activity and for future assessment of treatment response.

HISTOLOGY

Histologic evaluation of intestinal mucosa is essential for the diagnosis of IBD and can help differentiate between CD and UC. The endoscopist should separately and systematically obtain at least two biopsy specimens from each segment of the colon and ileum during a colonoscopy done for disease assessment.

- Ileum
- Right colon
- Transverse colon
- Left colon
- Sigmoid colon
- Rectum

Biopsies should be taken in inflamed and noninflamed areas to accurately assess disease distribution.[3,43] Colonoscopy underestimates the extent of disease when compared with histology, and the extent of colitis should be based on pathologic examination rather than only endoscopy.[2]

Biopsies can help differentiate IBD from other types of intestinal inflammation that may mimic the condition (see **Table 1**). In CD and UC, histology shows acute and chronic inflammation. Findings that suggest chronicity include crypt architectural distortion, Paneth cell metaplasia, pyloric gland metaplasia, basal plasmacytosis, and increased cellularity of the lamina propria.[54] Findings of chronicity are typically

Table 4
Simple endoscopic score for Crohn's disease

Variable	0	1	2	3
Size of ulcers	None	Aphthous ulcers (0.1–0.5 cm)	Large ulcers (0.5–2 cm)	Very large ulcers (>2 cm)
% Ulcerated surface	None	<10%	10%–30%	>30%
% Affected surface	None	<50%	50%–75%	>75%
Presence of narrowing	None	Single, can be passed	Multiple, can be passed	Impassable

Affected surface includes pseudopolyps, healed ulcers, frank erythema, edematous mucosa, ulcerations, and stenosis.
 Scored for each of five segments: ileum, right colon, transverse colon, left colon, and rectum.
 Data from Daperno M, D'Haens G, Van Assche G, et al. Development and validation of a new, simplified endoscopic activity score for Crohn's disease: the SES-CD. Gastrointest Endosc 2004;60(4):505–12.

absent in infectious colitis; other factors, such as length of symptomatology, infectious stool studies, and stains of the mucosa for infectious organisms, are important for making the correct diagnosis. At the time of colonoscopy, stool samples may also be taken and sent directly to the laboratory for common infections including *Clostridium difficile*. Similarly, there may be histologic clues to the presence of other types of intestinal inflammation, but clinical factors are a major determinant in the diagnosis.[11]

In patients with CD, granulomas are found on endoscopic biopsy in approximately 25% of specimens, with higher yield when taken around the edges of ulcers.[2,55] Because of the poor sensitivity of granulomas in intestinal biopsies, the presence of a granuloma is not required for a diagnosis. Additionally, granulomas are not specific for CD and are seen in other diseases, including intestinal tuberculosis, other infections, Behçet disease, sarcoidosis, chronic granulomatous disease, foreign body reaction, and diversion colitis.[11] In UC, a different type of loosely formed microgranuloma with pale foamy histiocytes is found adjacent to a damaged crypt, and this does not necessarily indicate a diagnosis of CD.[56] Well-formed epithelioid granulomas, away from the site of epithelial injury, support a diagnosis of CD.

The severity of histologic inflammation can be assessed using a grading system. More than 20 indices have been proposed for grading inflammation in UC, including the Harpaz score,[57,58] the Geboes score,[59] and the Nancy histologic index.[60] The Geboes score accounts for five grades of histologic inflammation, each with multiple subgrades.[59] Categories include the following:

- Structural/architectural changes (grade 0)
- Chronic inflammatory infiltrate (grade 1)
- Lamina propria neutrophils and eosinophils (grade 2)
- Neutrophils in epithelium (grade 3)
- Crypt destruction (grade 4)
- Erosion or ulceration (grade 5)

Recently, a simpler three descriptor index, the Nancy histologic index, has been validated for use in clinical practice and clinical trials, with good interobserver and intraobserver reliability and responsiveness to change. The severity of histologic inflammation is graded based on the presence of ulceration, acute inflammatory cell infiltrate, and chronic inflammatory infiltrate (**Fig. 5**).[60]

There are fewer histologic scoring indices for CD. The Colonic Global Histologic Disease Activity Score and Ileal Global Histologic Disease Activity Score have been used in the literature, and include assessment of the presence and extent of epithelial damage, architectural changes, infiltration of mononuclear cells in lamina propria, infiltration of polymorphonuclear cells in the lamina propria, polymorphonuclear cells in epithelium, erosions or ulceration, granulomas, and number of biopsy specimens affected. This scoring system is not commonly used in clinical practice.[61]

ASSESSMENT OF THE UPPER GASTROINTESTINAL TRACT

Esophagogastroduodenoscopy (EGD) can also be a useful tool in the initial diagnosis of IBD. Approximately 15% of patients with CD have involvement of their upper GI tract, more commonly in children.[3,9] Most of these patients also have disease in the lower GI tract. EGD is recommended in adult patients with upper GI symptoms and in all pediatric patients with suspicion for IBD.[3]

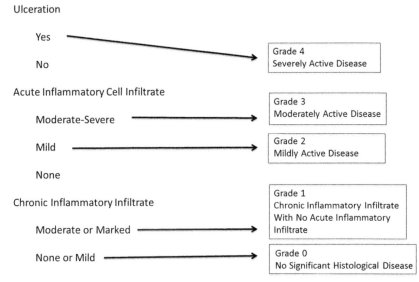

Fig. 5. Nancy histologic index. (*Data from* Marchal-Bressenot A, Salleron J, Boulagnon-Rombi C, et al. Development and validation of the Nancy histological index for UC. Gut 2015;1–7.)

In CD, the endoscopic appearance can include erythema, edema, aphthous ulcerations, and strictures in the esophagus, stomach, or duodenum. Biopsies from the stomach can show focal or patchy chronic inflammation, particularly *Helicobacter pylori*–negative focally active chronic gastritis. Biopsies from the duodenum can show intraepithelial lymphocytosis without villous atrophy, focal crypt distortion, and deformed and attenuated duodenal villi at times.[62,63] In upper GI tract CD, granulomas are found more commonly on histology, in up to 68% of biopsies.[3]

Patients with UC can also develop diffuse duodenitis, occurring on biopsy in up to 23% of children and up to 10% of adults.[64,65] Gastritis without aphthae can also be seen in patients with UC, and by itself, is not indicative of CD.

When performing EGD in suspected IBD with upper GI tract involvement, it is recommended to take at least two biopsies from the esophagus, stomach, and duodenum.[3] In one pediatric study, gastric antral biopsies with granulomatous inflammation changed the diagnosis to CD in 14% of patients.[66]

PROGNOSIS

The findings on initial colonoscopy may have prognostic implications for disease course. In Crohn's colitis, colonoscopy accurately predicts the severity of ulceration on the colectomy specimen.[67] Additionally, deep ulcerations on colonoscopy predict an increased rate of penetrating complications and surgery.[68]

There have been similar findings regarding colonoscopy in UC. Extensive deep ulcerations predict a high likelihood of surgery (**Fig. 6**), and severe endoscopic findings are consistent with deep extensive ulcerations on colectomy specimens.[69,70] Severe endoscopic lesions also predict nonresponse to medical therapy (odds ratio, 20.6; 95% confidence interval, 4.5–94.15).[71]

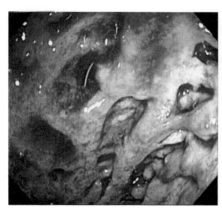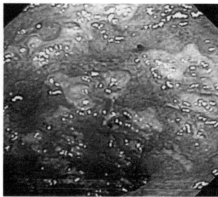

Fig. 6. Deep and well-like ulcerations in severe colitis.

SUMMARY

The first endoscopy in a patient with suspected IBD is essential for determining the correct diagnosis, and assessing the distribution and severity of disease. At the time of diagnosis, a full colonoscopy and ileoscopy should be performed when possible, with systematic biopsies from each segment, because macroscopic appearance often underestimates the histologic extent of disease. It is possible to distinguish between CD and UC in most patients, and the endoscopic features discussed in this review may assist in this delineation. It is important to obtain a correct assessment of disease characteristics and distribution before initiating therapy, because patchy healing can occur frequently. In the setting of severe deep colonic ulceration, endoscopic findings may have prognostic significance regarding response to medical therapy and need for surgery. In all patients with IBD, the initial endoscopic assessment and disease diagnosis have future implications for medical and surgical therapies, and for decisions regarding dysplasia surveillance. Therefore, it is important to take the opportunity for a complete and thorough evaluation of the ileum and colon before the initiation of medical therapy.

REFERENCES

1. Chutkan RK, Scherl E, Waye JD. Colonoscopy in inflammatory bowel disease. Gastrointest Endosc Clin N Am 2002;12:463–83.
2. Leighton JA, Shen B, Baron TH, et al, Standards of Practice Committee, American Society for Gastrointestinal Endoscopy. ASGE guideline: endoscopy in the diagnosis and treatment of inflammatory bowel disease. Gastrointest Endosc 2006; 63:558–65.
3. ASGE Standards of Practice Committee, Shergill AK, Lightdale JR, et al. The role of endoscopy in inflammatory bowel disease. Gastrointest Endosc 2015;81:1101–21.
4. Peyrin-Biroulet L, Loftus EV Jr, Tremaine WJ, et al. Perianal Crohn's disease findings other than fistulas in a population-based cohort. Inflamm Bowel Dis 2012;18:43–8.
5. Bonheur JL, Braunstein J, Korelitz BI, et al. Anal skin tags in inflammatory bowel disease: new observations and a clinical review. Inflamm Bowel Dis 2008;14: 1236–9.
6. Molnár T, Nagy F, Wittmann T. Anal skin tag: do not injure the elephants. J Clin Gastroenterol 2010;44:722.
7. Wolff BG, Culp CE, Beart RW Jr, et al. Anorectal Crohn's disease: a long-term perspective. Dis Colon Rectum 1985;28:709–11.

8. McClane SJ, Rombeau JL. Anorectal Crohn's disease. Surg Clin North Am 2001; 81:169–83.

9. Cosnes J, Gower-Rousseau C, Seksik P, et al. Epidemiology and natural history of inflammatory bowel diseases. Gastroenterology 2011;140:1785–94.

10. Nielsen OH, Vainer B, Rask-Madsen J. Non-IBD and noninfectious colitis. Nat Clin Pract Gastroenterol Hepatol 2008;5:28–39.

11. Sands BE. From symptom to diagnosis: clinical distinctions among various forms of intestinal inflammation. Gastroenterology 2004;126:1518–32.

12. Price AB. Pathology of drug-associated gastrointestinal disease. Br J Clin Pharmacol 2003;56:477–82.

13. Tursi A. Segmental colitis associated with diverticulosis: complication of diverticular disease or autonomous entity? Dig Dis Sci 2011;56:27–34.

14. Tursi A, Elisei W, Brandimarte G, et al. The endoscopic spectrum of segmental colitis associated with diverticulosis. Colorectal Dis 2010;12:464–70.

15. Pera A, Bellando P, Caldera D, et al. Colonoscopy in inflammatory bowel disease: diagnostic accuracy and proposal of an endoscopic score. Gastroenterology 1987;92:181–5.

16. Bernstein CN, Shanahan F, Anton PA, et al. Patchiness of mucosal inflammation in treated ulcerative colitis: a prospective study. Gastrointest Endosc 1995;42: 232–7.

17. Rubin DT, Rothe JA. The peri-appendiceal red patch in ulcerative colitis: review of the University of Chicago experience. Dig Dis Sci 2010;55:3495–501.

18. D'Haens G, Geboes K, Peeters M, et al. Patchy cecal inflammation associated with distal ulcerative colitis: a prospective endoscopic study. Am J Gastroenterol 1997;92:1275–9.

19. Yamagishi N, Iizuka B, Nakamura T, et al. Clinical and colonoscopic investigation of skipped periappendiceal lesions in ulcerative colitis. Scand J Gastroenterol 2002;37:177–82.

20. Byeon JS, Yang SK, Myung SJ, et al. Clinical course of distal ulcerative colitis in relation to appendiceal orifice inflammation status. Inflamm Bowel Dis 2005;11: 366–71.

21. Park SH, Loftus EV Jr, Yang SK. Appendiceal skip inflammation and ulcerative colitis. Dig Dis Sci 2014;59:2050–7.

22. Markowitz J, Kahn E, Grancher K, et al. Atypical rectosigmoid histology in children with newly diagnosed ulcerative colitis. Am J Gastroenterol 1993;88:2034–7.

23. Glickman JN, Bousvaros A, Farraye FA, et al. Pediatric patients with untreated ulcerative colitis may present initially with unusual morphologic findings. Am J Surg Pathol 2004;28:190–7.

24. Levine A, de Bie CI, Turner D, et al. EUROKIDS Porto IBD Working Group of ESPGHAN. Atypical disease phenotypes in pediatric ulcerative colitis: 5-year analyses of the EUROKIDS Registry. Inflamm Bowel Dis 2013;19:370–7.

25. Loftus EV Jr, Harewood GC, Loftus CG, et al. PSC-IBD: a unique form of inflammatory bowel disease associated with primary sclerosing cholangitis. Gut 2005; 54:91–6.

26. Park SH, Yang SK, Park SK, et al. Atypical distribution of inflammation in newly diagnosed ulcerative colitis is not rare. Can J Gastroenterol Hepatol 2014;28: 125–30.

27. Robert ME, Skacel M, Ullman T, et al. Patterns of colonic involvement at initial presentation in ulcerative colitis: a retrospective study of 46 newly diagnosed cases. Am J Clin Pathol 2004;122:94–9.

28. Rieder F, Zimmermann EM, Remzi FH, et al. Crohn's disease complicated by strictures: a systematic review. Gut 2013;62:1072–84.

29. Rieder F, Latella G, Magro F, et al. European Crohn's and Colitis Organisation topical review on prediction, diagnosis and management of fibrostenosing Crohn's disease. J Crohns Colitis 2016. [Epub ahead of print].

30. Gumaste V, Sachar DB, Greenstein AJ. Benign and malignant colorectal strictures in ulcerative colitis. Gut 1992;33:938–41.

31. Sonnenberg A, Genta RM. Epithelial dysplasia and cancer in IBD strictures. J Crohns Colitis 2015;9:769–75.

32. Friedman S, Rubin PH, Bodian C, et al. Screening and surveillance colonoscopy in chronic Crohn's colitis. Gastroenterology 2001;120:820–6.

33. Navaneethan U, Lourdusamy V, Njei B, et al. Endoscopic balloon dilation in the management of strictures in Crohn's disease: a systematic review and meta-analysis of non-randomized trials. Surg Endosc 2016. http://dx.doi.org/10.1007/s00464-016-4902-1.

34. Neilson LJ, Bevan R, Panter S, et al. Terminal ileal intubation and biopsy in routine colonoscopy practice. Expert Rev Gastroenterol Hepatol 2015;9:567–74.

35. Geboes K, Ectors N, D'Haens G, et al. Is ileoscopy with biopsy worthwhile in patients presenting with symptoms of inflammatory bowel disease? Am J Gastroenterol 1998;93:201–6.

36. Haskell H, Andrews CW Jr, Reddy SI, et al. Pathologic features and clinical significance of "backwash" ileitis in ulcerative colitis. Am J Surg Pathol 2005;29:1472.

37. Abdelrazeq AS, Wilson TR, Leitch DL, et al. Ileitis in ulcerative colitis: is it a backwash? Dis Colon Rectum 2005;48:2038.

38. Heuschen UA, Hinz U, Allemeyer EH, et al. Backwash ileitis is strongly associated with colorectal carcinoma in ulcerative colitis. Gastroenterology 2001;120:841–7.

39. Arrossi AV, Kariv Y, Bronner MP, et al. Backwash ileitis does not affect pouch outcome in patients with ulcerative colitis with restorative proctocolectomy. Clin Gastroenterol Hepatol 2011;9:981–8.

40. Devlin SM, Melmed GY, Irving PM, et al. Recommendations for quality colonoscopy reporting for patients with inflammatory bowel disease: results from a RAND Appropriateness Panel. Inflamm Bowel Dis 2016;22(6):1418–24.

41. Silverberg MS, Satsangi J, Ahmad T, et al. Toward an integrated clinical, molecular and serological classification of inflammatory bowel disease: report of a Working Party of the 2005 Montreal World Congress of Gastroenterology. Can J Gastroenterol 2005;19(Suppl A):5A–36A.

42. Spekhorst LM, Visschedijk MC, Alberts R, et al. Performance of the Montreal classification for inflammatory bowel diseases. World J Gastroenterol 2014;20:15374–81.

43. Nikolaus S, Schreiber S. Diagnostics of inflammatory bowel disease. Gastroenterology 2007 Nov;133:1670–89.

44. Mekhjian HS, Switz DM, Melnyk CS, et al. Clinical features and natural history of Crohn's disease. Gastroenterology 1979;77:898–906.

45. Daperno M, Comberlato M, Bossa F, et al. Inter-observer agreement in endoscopic scoring systems: preliminary report of an ongoing study from the Italian Group for Inflammatory Bowel Disease (IG-IBD). Dig Liver Dis 2014;46:969–73.

46. Ket SN, Palmer R, Travis S. Endoscopic disease activity in inflammatory bowel disease. Curr Gastroenterol Rep 2015;17:50.

47. Lobatón T, Bessissow T, De Hertogh G, et al. The Modified Mayo Endoscopic Score (MMES): a new index for the assessment of extension and severity of endoscopic activity in ulcerative colitis patients. J Crohns Colitis 2015;9:846–52.

48. Travis SP, Schnell D, Krzeski P, et al. Reliability and initial validation of the ulcerative colitis endoscopic index of severity. Gastroenterology 2013;145(5):987–95.

49. Ikeya K, Hanai H, Sugimoto K, et al. The ulcerative colitis endoscopic index of severity more accurately reflects clinical outcome and long-term prognosis than the Mayo endoscopic score. J Crohns Colitis 2016;10(3):286–95.

50. Walsh A, Palmer R, Travis S. Mucosal healing as a target of therapy for colonic inflammatory bowel disease and methods to score disease activity. Gastrointest Endosc Clin N Am 2014;24(3):367–78.

51. Mary JY, Modigliani R. Development and validation of an endoscopic index of the severity for Crohn's disease: a prospective multicentre study. Groupe d'Etudes Therapeutiques des Affections Inflammatoires du Tube Digestif (GETAID). Gut 1989;30:983–9.

52. Daperno M, D'Haens G, Van Assche G, et al. Development and validation of a new, simplified endoscopic activity score for Crohn's disease: the SES-CD. Gastrointest Endosc 2004;60(4):505–12.

53. Khanna R, Zou G, D'Haens G, et al. Reliability among central readers in the evaluation of endoscopic findings from patients with Crohn's disease. Gut 2015. http://dx.doi.org/10.1136/gutjnl-2014-308973.

54. Dundas SA, Dutton J, Skipworth P. Reliability of rectal biopsy in distinguishing between chronic inflammatory bowel disease and acute self-limited colitis. Histopathology 1997;31:60–6.

55. Pötzi R, Walgram M, Lochs H, et al. Diagnostic significance of endoscopic biopsy in Crohn's disease. Endoscopy 1989;21:60–2.

56. DeRoche TC, Xiao SY, Liu X. Histological evaluation in ulcerative colitis. Gastroenterol Rep 2014;2:178–92.

57. Fiel M, Qin L, Suriawinita A, et al. Histologic grading of disease activity in chronic IBD: inter- and intra-observer variation amongst pathologists with different levels of experience. Mod Pathol 2003;16:118A.

58. Bryant RV, Winer S, Travis SP, et al. Systematic review: histological remission in inflammatory bowel disease. Is 'complete' remission the new treatment paradigm? An IOIBD initiative. J Crohns Colitis 2014;8:1582–97.

59. Geboes K. A reproducible grading scale for histological assessment of inflammation in ulcerative colitis. Gut 2000;47:404–9.

60. Marchal-Bressenot A, Salleron J, Boulagnon-Rombi C, et al. Development and validation of the Nancy histological index for UC. Gut 2015. http://dx.doi.org/10.1136/gutjnl-2015-310187.

61. D'Haens GR, Geboes K, Peeters M, et al. Early lesions of recurrent Crohn's disease caused by infusion of intestinal contents in excluded ileum. Gastroenterology 1998;114:262–7.

62. Annunziata ML, Caviglia R, Papparella LG, et al. Upper gastrointestinal involvement of Crohn's disease: a prospective study on the role of upper endoscopy in the diagnostic work-up. Dig Dis Sci 2012;57:1618–23.

63. Patterson ER, Shmidt E, Oxentenko AS, et al. Normal villous architecture with increased intraepithelial lymphocytes: a duodenal manifestation of Crohn disease. Am J Clin Pathol 2015;143:445–50.

64. Tobin JM, Sinha B, Ramani P, et al. Upper gastrointestinal mucosal disease in pediatric Crohn disease and ulcerative colitis: a blinded, controlled study. J Pediatr Gastroenterol Nutr 2001;32:443–8.

65. Lin J, McKenna BJ, Appelman HD. Morphologic findings in upper gastrointestinal biopsies of patients with ulcerative colitis: a controlled study. Am J Surg Pathol 2010;34:1672–7.

66. Kundhal PS, Stormon MO, Zachos M, et al. Gastral antral biopsy in the differentiation of pediatric colitides. Am J Gastroenterol 2003;98:557–61.

67. Nahon S, Bouhnik Y, Lavergne-Slove A, et al. Colonoscopy accurately predicts the anatomical severity of colonic Crohn's disease attacks: correlation with findings from colectomy specimens. Am J Gastroenterol 2002;97:3102–7.

68. Allez M, Lemann M, Bonnet J, et al. Long term outcome of patients with active Crohn's disease exhibiting extensive and deep ulcerations at colonoscopy. Am J Gastroenterol 2002;97:947–53.

69. Carbonnel F, Lavergne A, Lemann M, et al. Colonoscopy of acute colitis. A safe and reliable tool for assessment of severity. Dig Dis Sci 1994;39:1550.

70. Allez M, Lémann M. Role of endoscopy in predicting the disease course in inflammatory bowel disease. World J Gastroenterol 2010;16:2626–32.

71. Daperno M, Sostegni R, Scaglione N, et al. Outcome of a conservative approach in severe ulcerative colitis. Dig Liver Dis 2004;36:21–8.

Capsule Endoscopy and Deep Enteroscopy in Irritable Bowel Disease

 CrossMark

Uri Kopylov, MD[a,b,*], Dan Carter, MD[a,b], Abraham Rami Eliakim, MD[a,b]

KEYWORDS

- Small-bowel video capsule endoscopy • Crohn's disease • Mucosal healing
- Classification • Postoperative recurrence • Device-assisted enteroscopy

KEY POINTS

- Capsule endoscopy and device-assisted enteroscopy provide thorough and accurate evaluation of the small bowel.
- Capsule endoscopy is a valuable tool for determination of disease location and phenotype, assessment of mucosal healing, and determination of postoperative recurrence.
- Device-assisted enteroscopy allows for histologic verification of the diagnosis and treatment of disease complications.

INTRODUCTION

The small bowel is involved in at least 70% of Crohn's disease (CD) patients, and in at least 30% of patients it involves the small bowel exclusively; the involved segments are frequently proximal to the terminal ileum and, thus, are inaccessible to standard ileocolonoscopic evaluation.[1] Video capsule endoscopy and device-assisted enteroscopy (DAE) have greatly expanded the ability to diagnose small-bowel pathologic conditions. Small-bowel capsule endoscopy (SBCE) (Given Imaging, Yokneam, Israel) has been available for clinical use since its authority's approval in the United States and Europe in 2001.[2] Several other manufacturers released their versions of the device since, and the basic operational principals are similar across models.[3] A growing body of evidence supports the use of SBCE for phenotyping, assessing severity and prognosis, and monitoring treatment in small-bowel CD, turning SBCE into a valuable decision-supporting tool. DAE incorporates a few diagnostic modalities for endoscopic endoluminal evaluation necessitating assisted progression, including push enteroscopy, single and double balloon enteroscopy, spiral enteroscopy,

[a] Department of Gastroenterology, Sheba Medical Center, Tel Hashomer 5265601, Israel;
[b] Sackler School of Medicine, Tel Aviv University, Tel Aviv 6910302, Israel
* Corresponding author. Department of Gastroenterology, Sheba Medical Center, Tel Hashomer, Israel.
E-mail address: ukopylov@gmail.com

Gastrointest Endoscopy Clin N Am 26 (2016) 611–627
http://dx.doi.org/10.1016/j.giec.2016.06.007
1052-5157/16/© 2016 Elsevier Inc. All rights reserved.

balloon-guided endoscopy, or intraoperative enteroscopy (**Fig. 1**). DAE enables histopathologic confirmation when other modalities such as ileocolonoscopy, SBCE, and cross-sectional imaging are inconclusive and also allows for therapeutic intervention.[4] The applications of video capsule endoscopy and DAE in established small-bowel CD are reviewed below.

DIAGNOSIS OF CROHN'S DISEASE BY CAPSULE ENDOSCOPY
Characteristic Endoscopic Findings

Several SBCE findings are frequently associated with CD: aphthous lesions, serpiginous, linear or deep ulcerations, and mucosal edema[5] (see **Fig. 1**). However, these findings are neither pathognomonic nor specific to CD. Some minor small-bowel lesions may be found in up to 10% of normal subjects,[6] but the most common mimickers of small-bowel CD are nonsteroidal anti-inflammatory medication (NSAID)-induced enteropathy, which may appear after a short exposure[7,8] Avoidance of NSAIDs for at least 1 month before SBCE examination is, therefore, mandatory for patients undergoing SBCE for suspected CD.[9]

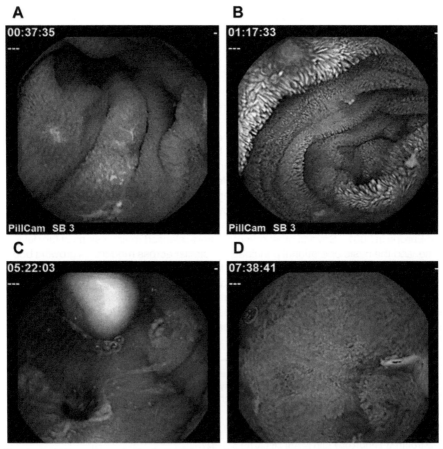

Fig. 1. Capsule endoscopy findings characteristic of CD. (A, B) Ulcerations. (C) Ulcerated stricture. (D) Mucosal edema.

Endoscopic/Diagnostic Scores

Several diagnostic criteria were used for diagnosis of CD on SBCE (**Table 1**). Earlier studies by Mow and colleagues[10] required detection of ≥3 ulcers to fulfill the criteria of definite diagnosis of CD. This definition was replaced by more stringent criteria. Two endoscopic inflammatory scores are currently available for diagnosis and monitoring of CD or other small-bowel inflammation. The Lewis score[11] was designed for quantification of small-bowel inflammation. This score divides the small bowel into 3 tertiles (identified by truncation of the small-bowel transit time) and assigns points to various findings (mucosal edema, ulcers, strictures) characteristic for CD in each of the tertiles, correcting for severity and extent of the findings. The Lewis score is incorporated in the software of the Medtronic/Given Imaging device (the RAPID software). A score less than 135 designates a normal small bowel, a score of 135 to 790 is considered mild to moderate inflammation, and a score ≥790 defines moderate-to-severe inflammation.[11] An additional score known as Capsule Endoscopy Crohn's Disease Activity Index (CECDAI) is also available.[12] This score divides the small bowel in 2 segments and incorporates the degree of inflammation, extent of disease, and strictures in both.[13] A significant correlation between the Lewis score and CECDAI was reported.[14] Both of these scores have been validated. The Lewis score is easy and user friendly as it is incorporated in the software and was also found to have better correlation with fecal calprotectin.[14]

Small-Bowel Capsule Endoscopy Versus Other Modalities for the Diagnosis of Crohn's Disease

SBCE has been repeatedly compared with other diagnostic modalities for detection of CD, such as small-bowel follow-through, computed tomography enterography (CTE), and magnetic resonance enterography (MRE). The superiority of SBCE diagnostic yield over small-bowel follow-through, CTE, and ileocolonoscopy was repeatedly demonstrated.[15–20] Despite the overall comparable accuracy of SBCE and MRE for detection of CD,[19] there are several distinctive advantages and weaknesses to each modality. MRE is naturally superior for detection of penetrating and other extraluminal complications. However, its sensitivity for detection of mild mucosal inflammation is significantly inferior to that of SBCE.[21] Moreover, the accuracy of MRE for detection of proximal small-bowel disease is poor.[22] Jensen and colleagues[23] reported that proximal small-bowel CD was detected in 18 of 93 patients by SBCE compared with 2 and 6 patients using MRE or CTE, respectively (P<.05). Moreover, the acceptability and willingness of patients to repeat the procedure is significantly higher for SBCE compared with MRE,[24] as bowel preparation for SBCE is not mandatory.[25]

Small-Bowel Capsule Endoscopy in Established Crohn's Disease

There are several potential applications for SBCE in patients with established CD. The main applications of capsule endoscopy in established CD include the following:

- Assessment of disease extent, severity and, thus, prognosis
- Evaluation of mucosal healing
- Evaluation of postoperative recurrence

Disease Reclassification and Prognosis

Disease phenotype (both location and behavior) impacts the long-term prognosis and the treatment strategy.[1] Patients with extensive/proximal small-bowel disease relapse sooner and are more prone to have surgery.[26,27] The importance of proximal small-bowel disease is reflected in the recently published pediatric Paris classification of

Table 1
Comparison of 2 capsule endoscopy scoring indices for quantification of mucosal inflammation

Parameter	Lewis Score[11]			CECDAI[12]	
	Number/Quality	Longitudinal Extent	Descriptors		
Villous appearance	Normal/edematous	Short segment/long segment/whole tertile	Single/patchy/diffuse	Inflammation score	None to large ulcer (>2 cm)
Ulceration	None/single/few/multiple	Short segment/long segment/whole tertile	<25%, 25%–50%, 50>%	Extent of disease	No disease to diffuse
Stricture	None/single/few/multiple	Ulcerated/nonulcerated	Traversed/nontraversed	Stricture score	None to complete obstruction
Small-bowel segmentation	Tertiles (strictures for the length of the examination)			Proximal to distal small bowel	
Score	<135, normal or clinically insignificant inflammation 135–790, mild inflammation >790, moderate-to-severe inflammation.			0 (normal examination) –26 (severe inflammation)	

CD[28]; however, a similar change was not yet adopted in the adult Montreal classification.[29] SBCE is capable of detecting active disease in previously unknown locations. Although MRE was not sensitive for detection of jejunal and proximal ileal CD, capsule endoscopy detected proximal lesions in more than 50% of patients with established small-bowel CD.[30] In patients with a diagnosis of exclusively colonic CD, small-bowel involvement was diagnosed in 25.6% of patients in a recent large retrospective study.[31] Phenotype changes can also be detected by SBCE. Although patients with severe fibrostenotic phenotype are usually not given an SBCE or they undergo a patency capsule procedure or cross-sectional imaging to rule out stricturing disease before an SBCE,[9] previously unknown fibrostenotic disease can still be detected via SBCE in up to 11% of the patients.[30]

SBCE is useful in establishment of the final diagnosis in patients with undetermined inflammatory bowel disease (IBD). Colonic inflammatory bowel disease cannot be classified as CD or ulcerative colitis using current ileocolonoscopic and pathologic criteria in 10% to 15% of the patients[32] and thus is named *IBD unclassified*. However, up to 30% of disease will be reclassified as CD during the course of the follow-up.[33] Ascertainment of the diagnosis is especially important in severe cases requiring a surgical intervention, as rates of chronic pouchitis and pouch failure after ileal pouch-anal anastomosis are significantly higher in patients with CD.[34] Mow and colleagues[10] have described 22 patients with either isolated colitis or chronic symptoms following ileal pouch-anal anastomosis that had prior unremarkable small-bowel radiography. Multiple ulcerations (3 or more) were identified in 59% of these patients. Mehdizadeh and colleagues[35] described 120 patients with a history of ulcerative colitis or IBD unclassified who underwent SBCE. Findings consistent with small-bowel CD were seen in 15.8% of the patients.

Evaluation of Mucosal Healing

The leading treatment paradigm in IBD has shifted in the last years from merely controlling symptoms to reversing the underlying inflammation.[36–39] The concept of deep or stable remission, defined as a combination of clinical remission and mucosal healing, is an emerging treatment goal in clinical trials.[40] However, most current knowledge pertains to mucosal healing in the colon and the terminal ileum that does not necessarily correlate with the degree of inflammation in the proximal small bowel.[41] Determining what actually constitutes "small-bowel mucosal healing" is a crucial issue if this goal is to be adapted in future clinical trials or routine clinical practice. Recently, the Lewis score, originally developed to distinguish inflammatory from noninflammatory findings,[11] was validated for monitoring of small-bowel mucosal healing in CD.[42] A cutoff value of 135, consistent with the original value representing normal small bowel, was confirmed as a reasonable definition of mucosal healing in this large-scale Portuguese study.[42] Since then, several other studies adopted this definition.[14,22,30] The alternative diagnostic score (CECDAI) does not address a specific definition of mucosal healing; however, in a recent study that evaluated a correlation between the scores, the Lewis score value of 135 was consistent with a CECDAI of 3.8.[14]

To date, only some studies addressed monitoring of mucosal healing by SBCE in CD, and some additional studies are ongoing. A small prospective study evaluated monitoring of mucosal healing with SBCE performed before and after treatment for acute CD flare-up.[43] Forty patients with CD flares were included in the study, and all responded within 4 to 8 weeks of treatment. A significant improvement was seen in a subgroup of patients treated with corticosteroids combined with immunomodulators or biologics.

Two recent studies evaluated mucosal healing in CD patients taking immunomodulators or biologics after 12[44] or 52 weeks of therapy,[45] respectively. The investigators used the CECDAI score and defined complete mucosal healing as absence of ulcers, whereas mild disease was defined as CECDAI less than 3.5 and moderate-to-severe disease as CECDAI $\geq$5.8. The study cohort included 37 patients with established CD, 84% of who were started on adalimumab and the rest on azathioprine treatment. In the initial assessment, moderate-to-severe disease activity was detected in 67% of the patients and mild-to-moderate disease in 33%. After 12 weeks, clinical remission was achieved by 54% of the patients, and a significant decrease in both C-reactive protein (CRP) and fecal calprotectin was achieved as well. However, the mucosal response was significantly more modest; significant CECDAI improvement was seen in only 27% of the patients, whereas none achieved complete mucosal healing.[44] By week 52, 42% of the patients achieved complete mucosal healing that was also paralleled by clinical and biochemical remission.

A recent prospective study evaluated the prevalence of small-bowel mucosal healing using SBCE in patients with established small-bowel disease. Small-bowel mucosal healing was seen in 8 of 52 (15.4%) patients in clinical remission. Moderate-to-severe small-bowel inflammation was seen in 11 of 52 (21.1%) patients in clinical remission and in 1 of 21 (4.7%) of patients in clinical and biomarker remission. Only 7 of 52 (13.5%) patients were in deep remission.[22] The long-term impact of a low-grade (Lewis score, 135–790) small-bowel inflammation on the long-term prognosis and the risk of complications are still to be determined.

To date, a single industry–funded, small-scale, phase 2 study from Israel[46] that used serial SBCE follow-up within the setup of a clinical trial was published. No correlation between the Lewis score and clinical parameters (CDAI, Inflammatory Bowel Disease Questionnaire) or biomarkers was seen in this small study; the procedure itself was safe and well tolerated.[46] These data suggest that SBCE may be used as a less-invasive yet accurate way to look at mucosal healing in small-bowel CD, especially when the proximal small intestine is involved.

Monitoring of Postoperative Crohn's Disease Recurrence

Endoscopic recurrence of small-bowel CD in the neo-terminal ileum after surgical resection is frequent without secondary preventive measures and is seen in 73% to 93% of the patients within 1 year of surgery.[47,48] The current paradigm of postoperative surveillance and treatment is based on early and intensive endoscopic surveillance with aggressive treatment of high-risk patients[49,50] SBCE may provide a comprehensive and safe alternative to repeated ileo-colonoscopies in these patients and may also reveal active disease in the proximal small bowel, potentially necessitating earlier and more aggressive intervention. The Rutgeerts score is frequently used to quantify postoperative small-bowel inflammatory findings; higher scores are associated with a rapid progression to clinical relapse.[47] Bourreille and colleagues[51] evaluated the accuracy of SBCE versus ileocolonoscopy for detection of postoperative recurrence. In this cohort, recurrence occurred in 68% of the patients enrolled within 32 months from surgery. The sensitivity of SBCE was 62% to 76% and the specificity was 90% to 100%. The severity of lesions as assessed by both methodologies correlated significantly ($P<.05$).[51] In an additional study that included 24 postoperative CD patients, neo-terminal ileum recurrence defined as Rutgeerts score greater than 2 was shown by ileocolonoscopy in 25% of patients and by capsule endoscopy in 62%. Capsule endoscopy detected proximal SB lesions inaccessible by ileocolonoscopy in 13 patients.[52]

Correlation Between Endoscopic Findings and Inflammatory Biomarkers

Inflammatory biomarkers have a pivotal role in noninvasive management of CD. CRP is still probably the most available and used biomarker; however, almost 30% of CD patients with active disease do not have elevate CRP levels.[53] Fecal calprotectin (FCP) is significantly more sensitive than CRP for detection of mucosal inflammation in CD.[54] Because of cost considerations, it is tempting to use FCP as a triage tool guiding selection of patients for SBCE. However, it seems that the correlation of FCP levels with small-bowel inflammation as detected by SBCE in CD is not as strong as it is in the colon.[53] A recent meta-analysis that pooled the results of 7 studies reporting on SBCE findings and calprotectin levels, found a strong correlation between the 2 for all evaluated cutoffs (50, 100, and 200 μg/g). For studies including patients with suspected CD only, the overall accuracy for FC cutoff of 50 μg/g was excellent (sensitivity, 0.89; specificity, 0.55; and a negative predictive value of 91.8%). In patients with established CD, the likelihood of detection of a low-degree mucosal inflammation (Lewis score, 135–790) was almost 62% when a cutoff value of 100 μg/g was used for FC; however, severe inflammation (Lewis score >790) was rare (4.7%).[22]

Therapeutic Yield of Small-Bowel Capsule Endoscopy in Established Crohn's Disease

In known CD patients, SBCE is usually performed in routine clinical practice when a clinical dilemma arises. The capsule's results frequently lead to a change in therapy. In the largest case series of established CD patients evaluated with SBCE to date, a change in therapeutic management was suggested in 52.3% of 187 included patients, mainly escalation of anti-inflammatory therapy in 82.5% of the patients who required a change in therapy.[55]

Safety Considerations

The main complication of SBCE is capsule retention, defined as a failure to excrete the capsule requiring directed medical, endoscopic, or surgical intervention (**Fig. 2**).[56]

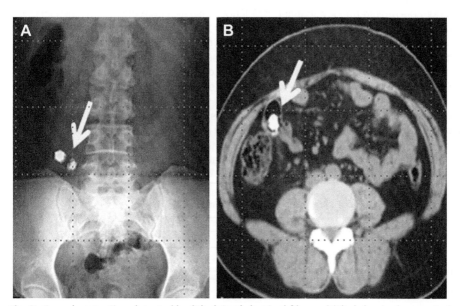

Fig. 2. Capsule retention detected by (*A*) plain abdominal film and (*B*) abdominal computed tomography scan. The retained capsule is marked by the *arrows*.

The risk of capsule retention is increased in patients with known small-bowel strictures, extensive small-bowel CD, history of small-bowel obstruction, and previous abdominal surgery[3] (**Table 2**). The risk of capsule retention in patients with established CD was reported to be as high as 13%,[10,57] however, in more recent series that verified small-bowel patency before performing SBCE, the risk of retention was much lower (1.5%–7.5%).[3,27,31,44–46,58] In the largest case series reported to date (406 patients), the rate of SBCE retention was 2.3%.[59] Capsule retention is usually uneventful but may present with symptoms of partial or complete bowel obstruction. In approximately half of the cases, the capsule is excreted spontaneously or after a short course of corticosteroids; if this method fails, the capsule can be extracted by DAE or surgically.[31,60] In rare cases, the capsule may remain in the small bowel or the colon without causing any symptoms for weeks or months.[61] It is unclear whether these cases merit endoscopic or surgical procedures or what the optimal timing is of such intervention.

PATENCY CAPSULE

Because of the increased risk of capsule retention in patients with CD, current European Crohn's and Colitis Organisation/European Society of Gastrointestinal Endoscopy guidelines recommend to assess small-bowel patency either via the use of a patency capsule or cross-sectional imaging before SBCE examination in patients with established CD.[4] For patients evaluated for suspected CD, routine patency evaluation is not recommended unless other risk factors (eg, history of abdominal surgery/radiation, obstructive symptoms) exist.

The patency capsule (PC; Agile, Given Imaging, Yokneam, Israel) is a nondiagnostic capsule of the same shape and dimensions as the diagnostic capsule. It is constructed of cellophane with wax plugs at either end and is filled with lactose mixed with 10% barium. The wax plugs are hollow and allow the enteric content to admix with the PC body leading to capsule disintegration (**Fig. 3**).[62] Because of the high barium content, the capsule remains radiopaque until dissolution; it can be detected by radiography or a portable radiofrequency scanner.[63–65] If not eliminated from the gastrointestinal tract, the patency capsule starts to disintegrate after 30 hours. When the patency capsule is successfully excreted or is not detectable with a radiofrequency scanner or plain abdominal radiography in the small bowel 30 hours after ingestion, it is safe to perform the diagnostic SBCE examination. The excretion rate of the patency capsule varies between 45% and 93%,[63,65–68] depending on patient selection. Diagnostic capsule retention may still occur after timely excretion of the PC; however, this is rare.[59] Performance of diagnostic SBCE despite a positive PC test result is associated with a high risk (11%) of capsule retention.[59] Cross-sectional imaging is an alternative to PC for establishment of small-bowel patency; comparative data for the 2 modalities are scarce; however, it seems that cross-sectional imaging overestimates the risk of retention.[69]

Table 2	
The risk of retention of SBCE by in different indications	
Overall	1.4%
Suspected CD	1.4%
Established CD	1.7%–7.5%
Obscure gastrointestinal bleeding	<5%
Suspected small-bowel obstruction	21%

Adapted from Eliakim R. Videocapsule endoscopy of the small bowel. Curr Opin Gastroenterol 2013;29:133–9.

A   **B**

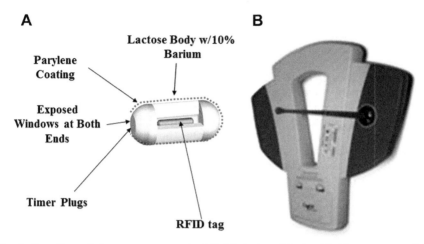

Lactose Body w/10% Barium

Parylene Coating

Exposed Windows at Both Ends

Timer Plugs

RFID tag

Fig. 3. Excretion of the patency capsule. (*A*) PC design. (*B*) Hand-held scanner used for assessment of PC elimination from the small bowel.

The main complication of patency capsule is mild abdominal pain, occurring in about 20% of the patients. Several dozens of cases of partial or complete small-bowel obstruction were reported in the literature, mainly with the first-generation capsule; the largest case series included 20 cases of obstruction of 1615 PC procedures performed.[70] In most cases, the obstruction resolved spontaneously or after a short course of corticosteroids.

DEVICE-ASSISTED ENTEROSCOPY IN CROHN'S DISEASE

The main indications for the use of DAE in small-bowel CD are summarized in **Box 1**. The diagnostic yield of DAE in suspected CD ranges between 25% and 70%, increasing when guided by a previous positive SBCE examination.[71] Other important indications for the use of DAE in CD include directed endoscopic therapy in cases of small-bowel strictures or bleeding and for retained capsule retrieval. Small-bowel strictures occur in 25% of CD patients,[72] mainly at the site of the surgical anastomosis in the terminal ileum or at the ileocecal valve. Possible therapeutic options include pneumatic dilatation using the through-the-scope balloons, hemostasis, local injection of steroids and immunomodulatory drugs, polypectomy, and the insertion of metallic and biodegradable stents.[73–76] When performing balloon dilatation of strictures, one typically uses balloons between 5 and 8 cm in length and up to 25 mm in diameter. The reported technical success rates reach 90%, with only 3% having complications.[77] A stricture length of ≤ 4 cm has been associated with better dilatation

---

Box 1
Main indication for the use of DAE in small-bowel CD

A. Histopathologic confirmation of CD when conventional studies are inconclusive and histologic diagnosis would alter disease management

B. Directed endoscopic therapy for small-bowel strictures and bleeding

C. Withdrawal of retained small-bowel capsule after failure of prior medical therapy

outcome,[78] whereas gastroduodenal strictures, which are of more fibrotic nature, may not benefit from dilatation.[79]

Push enteroscopy is used for examination of proximal small bowel, with the advantage of not requiring special equipment or training. The average depth of intubation at push enteroscopy using an enteroscope is reported to be approximately 25 to 63 cm beyond the ligament of Treitz, 46 to 80 cm for enteroscopy that uses an overtube, and 45 to 60 cm using a colonoscope.[80–82] Deeper small bowel intubation can be achieved with the use of balloon-assisted systems, which can be introduced to the small bowel via the oral (antegrade) or anal (retrograde) route. The systems consist of the double balloon enteroscope (DBE) (Fujinon Inc, Saitama, Japan) or the single balloon enteroscope (SBE) (Olympus Corporation, Tokyo, Japan) (**Fig. 4**). Deep small bowel intubation is achieved by a series of advancement cycles that use the push-and-pull technique, folding the bowel onto the endoscope. DBE consists of an enteroscope and an overtube, both of which have balloons at their distal ends. The SBE has an enteroscope and an overtube, with a balloon only on the overtube. Both enteroscopes have a working length of 200 cm. DBE has an overtube length of 140 cm and an outer diameter of 9.4 mm, whereas SBE has an overtube of 132 cm and an outer diameter of 9.8 mm (**Table 3**). Deep small-bowel intubations of up to 240 to 360 cm antegrade and

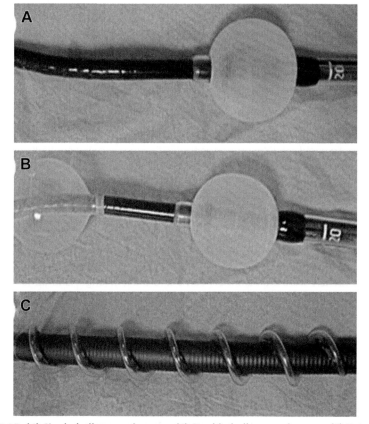

Fig. 4. DAE. (*A*) Single balloon endoscope. (*B*) Double balloon endoscope. (*C*) Spiral endoscope. (*Adapted from* Dye CE, Gaffney RR, Dykes TM, et al. Endoscopic and radiographic evaluation of the small bowel in 2012. Am J Med 2012;125(12):1228.e1-e12.)

Table 3
Comparison between the different available DAE

	Double Balloon	Single Balloon	Spiral Enteroscopy	On-Demand Balloon
System	Working length, 200 cm; outer diameter, 9.4 mm; overtube length, 140 cm	Working length, 200 cm; outer diameter, 9.8 mm; overtube length, 132 cm	A spiral-shaped overtube 118 cm long; the hollow spiral are 5.5 mm high and 22 cm long	Working length of 350 cm with a balloon diameter of 40 mm Minimum working channel diameter 3.8 mm
Depth of insertion (antegrade)	240–360 cm	Similar to DBE	176–262 cm (from the ligament of Treitz)	Unknown
Depth of insertion (retrograde)	102–140 cm	Similar to DBE	Limited ileoscopy	Unknown
Total enteroscopy	Possible (16%–86%)	Possible (0%–22%)	Not possible	Not possible
Therapeutic intervention	Possible	Possible	Possible	Possible
Diagnostic yield	60%–80%	37%–62%	33%	Unknown
Complication rate	0.8%–4%	Similar to DBE	0.3%; perforation rate, 0.27%	Unknown

102 to 140 cm retrograde are possible, although complete evaluation of the small bowel was reported only in 16% to 86%.[83,84] A range of accessories allow tissue sampling and therapeutic procedures, enabling the acquisition of tissue biopsies and the performance of various therapeutic procedures as hemostasis, polypectomy, dilation, and stent placement. The main disadvantage of balloon-assisted enteroscopy results from the invasive and complex nature of the procedure that necessitates performance by experienced and well-trained endoscopists and by the long duration of the procedure and the requirement for deep sedation when performing the examination via an antegrade approach. The main complications reported are ileus, pancreatitis, and perforations, which are reported in 0.8% of the diagnostic procedures and in up to 4% in the therapeutic procedures (see **Table 3**).[85,86] Spiral enteroscopy achieves deep small-bowel anterograde intubation using a single-use overtube (Endo-Ease Discovery SB; Spirus Medical, Stoughton, MA) (see **Fig. 1**). The overtube has helical spirals at its distal end and rotates independently from the enteroscope. It is 118 cm long with a locking device on the proximal end. This system is limited for the use of enteroscopes of less than 9.4 mm in diameter. There is also an overtube for a rectal approach called the Endo-Ease Vista Retrograde (Spirus Medical), which can be used for limited ileoscopy. The reported depth of insertion is deeper, 176 to 262 cm from the ligament of Treitz.[87] The performance of diagnostic and therapeutic procedures, including biopsy, hemostasis, and polypectomy, is possible. Major complications were reported in 0.3%, with small-bowel perforation and pneumoperitoneum being the most common complications (see **Table 3**). The NaviAid AB device (SMART Medical Systems Ltd, Ra'anana, Israel) is a newer on-demand balloon system, consisting of a disposable balloon component that is advanced through the working channel of a conventional colonoscope (NaviAid AB and NaviAid ABC) and an air supply unit.[4,88] The NaviAid AB has a working length of 350 cm with a balloon diameter of 40 mm. The balloon is inflated to anchor in the intestine, and a repetitive push-pull technique is performed, with the endoscope sliding over the guiding catheter to the balloon inflated in the distal small bowel. Once therapeutic intervention is needed, the balloon catheter is removed, followed by reinstitution for further advancement after the intervention procedure is ended.

SUMMARY

Capsule endoscopy allows accurate and safe evaluation of the small bowel in patients with CD. This modality has significantly expanded understanding of the true inflammatory burden of CD outside the colon and the terminal ileum. Small-bowel mucosal healing is an emerging concept in CD monitoring and a potential therapeutic goal for both clinical trials and routine practice. DAE allows for evaluation and therapeutic interventions for CD complications and may frequently alleviate the need for surgery in complicated cases.

REFERENCES

1. Cosnes J, Gower-Rousseau C, Seksik P, et al. Epidemiology and natural history of inflammatory bowel diseases. Gastroenterology 2011;140:1785–94.
2. Nakamura T, Terano A. Capsule endoscopy: past, present, and future. J Gastroenterol 2008;43:93–9.
3. Eliakim R. Video capsule endoscopy of the small bowel. Curr Opin Gastroenterol 2013;29:133–9.
4. Pennazio M, Spada C, Eliakim R, et al. Small-bowel capsule endoscopy and device-assisted enteroscopy for diagnosis and treatment of small-bowel

disorders: European Society of Gastrointestinal Endoscopy (ESGE) Clinical Guideline. Endoscopy 2015;47:352–86.

5. Bourreille A, Ignjatovic A, Aabakken L, et al. Role of small-bowel endoscopy in the management of patients with inflammatory bowel disease: an international OMED-ECCO consensus. Endoscopy 2009;41:618–37.

6. Bar-Meir S. Review article: capsule endoscopy - are all small intestinal lesions Crohn's disease? Aliment Pharmacol Ther 2006;24(Suppl 3):19–21.

7. Graham DY, Opekun AR, Willingham FF, et al. Visible small-intestinal mucosal injury in chronic NSAID users. Clin Gastroenterol Hepatol 2005;3:55–9.

8. Maiden L, Thjoleifsson B, Seigal A, et al. Long-term effects of nonsteroidal anti-inflammatory drugs and cyclooxygenase-2 selective agents on the small bowel: a cross-sectional capsule enteroscopy study. Clin Gastroenterol Hepatol 2007;5: 1040–5.

9. Annese V, Daperno M, Rutter MD, et al. European evidence based consensus for endoscopy in inflammatory bowel disease. J Crohns Colitis 2013;7:982–1018.

10. Mow WS, Lo SK, Targan SR, et al. Initial experience with wireless capsule entero-scopy in the diagnosis and management of inflammatory bowel disease. Clin Gastroenterol Hepatol 2004;2:31–40.

11. Gralnek IM, Defranchis R, Seidman E, et al. Development of a capsule endos-copy scoring index for small bowel mucosal inflammatory change. Aliment Phar-macol Ther 2008;27:146–54.

12. Niv Y, Ilani S, Levi Z, et al. Validation of the Capsule Endoscopy Crohn's Disease Activity Index (CECDAI or Niv score): a multicenter prospective study. Endoscopy 2012;44:21–6.

13. Rosa B, Moreira MJ, Rebelo A, et al. Lewis Score: a useful clinical tool for patients with suspected Crohn's Disease submitted to capsule endoscopy. J Crohns Colitis 2012;6:692–7.

14. Koulaouzidis A, Douglas S, Plevris JN. Lewis score correlates more closely with fecal calprotectin than Capsule Endoscopy Crohn's Disease Activity Index. Dig Dis Sci 2012;57:987–93.

15. de Melo SW Jr, Di Palma JA. The role of capsule endoscopy in evaluating inflam-matory bowel disease. Gastroenterol Clin North Am 2012;41:315–23.

16. Marmo R, Rotondano G, Piscopo R, et al. Meta-analysis: capsule enteroscopy vs. conventional modalities in diagnosis of small bowel diseases. Aliment Pharmacol Ther 2005;22:595–604.

17. Marmo R, Rotondano G, Piscopo R, et al. Capsule endoscopy versus enterocly-sis in the detection of small-bowel involvement in Crohn's disease: a prospective trial. Clin Gastroenterol Hepatol 2005;3:772–6.

18. Triester SL, Leighton JA, Leontiadis GI, et al. A meta-analysis of the yield of capsule endoscopy compared to other diagnostic modalities in patients with non-stricturing small bowel Crohn's disease. Am J Gastroenterol 2006;101: 954–64.

19. Dionisio PM, Gurudu SR, Leighton JA, et al. Capsule endoscopy has a signifi-cantly higher diagnostic yield in patients with suspected and established small-bowel Crohn's disease: a meta-analysis. Am J Gastroenterol 2010;105: 1240–8 [quiz: 1249].

20. Jensen MD, Kjeldsen J, Rafaelsen SR, et al. Diagnostic accuracies of MR enterography and CT enterography in symptomatic Crohn's disease. Scand J Gastroenterol 2011;46:1449–57.

21. Kopylov U, Klang E, Yablecovitch E, et al. Magnetic resonance enterography versus capsule endoscopy activity indices for quantification of small bowel

inflammation in Crohn's disease. Therap Adv Gastroenterol 2016. [Epub ahead of print].

22. Kopylov U, Yablecovitch D, Lahat A, et al. Detection of small bowel mucosal healing and deep remission in patients with known small bowel Crohn's disease using biomarkers, capsule endoscopy, and imaging. Am J Gastroenterol 2015;110: 1316–23.

23. Jensen MD, Nathan T, Rafaelsen SR, et al. Diagnostic accuracy of capsule endoscopy for small bowel Crohn's disease is superior to that of MR enterography or CT enterography. Clin Gastroenterol Hepatol 2011;9:124–9.

24. Lahat A, Kopylov U, Amitai MM, et al. Magnetic resonance enterography or video capsule endoscopy – what do Crohn's disease patients prefer? Patient Prefer Adherence 2016;10:1043–50.

25. Klein A, Dashkovsky M, Gralnek I, et al. Bowel preparation in "real-life" small bowel capsule endoscopy: a two-center experience. Ann Gastroenterol 2016; 29:196–200.

26. Park SK, Yang SK, Park SH, et al. Long-term prognosis of the jejunal involvement of Crohn's disease. J Clin Gastroenterol 2013;47:400–8.

27. Flamant M, Trang C, Maillard O, et al. The prevalence and outcome of jejunal lesions visualized by small bowel capsule endoscopy in Crohn's disease. Inflamm Bowel Dis 2013;19:1390–6.

28. Levine A, Griffiths A, Markowitz J, et al. Pediatric modification of the Montreal classification for inflammatory bowel disease: the Paris classification. Inflamm Bowel Dis 2011;17:1314–21.

29. Satsangi J, Silverberg MS, Vermeire S, et al. The Montreal classification of inflammatory bowel disease: controversies, consensus, and implications. Gut 2006;55: 749–53.

30. Greener T, Klang E, Yablecovitch D, et al. The impact of magnetic resonance enterography and capsule endoscopy on the re-classification of disease in patients with known Crohn's Disease: a prospective Israeli IBD Research Nucleus (IIRN) Study. J Crohns Colitis 2016;10(5):525–31.

31. Kopylov U, Nemeth A, Koulaouzidis A, et al. Small bowel capsule endoscopy in the management of established Crohn's disease: clinical impact, safety, and correlation with inflammatory biomarkers. Inflamm Bowel Dis 2015;21:93–100.

32. Guindi M, Riddell RH. Indeterminate colitis. J Clin Pathol 2004;57:1233–44.

33. Eliakim R. The impact of wireless capsule endoscopy on gastrointestinal diseases. South Med J 2007;100:235–6.

34. Fazio VW, Ziv Y, Church JM, et al. Ileal pouch-anal anastomoses complications and function in 1005 patients. Ann Surg 1995;222:120–7.

35. Mehdizadeh S, Chen G, Enayati PJ, et al. Diagnostic yield of capsule endoscopy in ulcerative colitis and inflammatory bowel disease of unclassified type (IBDU). Endoscopy 2008;40:30–5.

36. Vuitton L, Marteau P, Sandborn WJ, et al. IOIBD technical review on endoscopic indices for Crohn's disease clinical trials. Gut 2015. [Epub ahead of print].

37. Pineton de Chambrun G, Blanc P, Peyrin-Biroulet L. Current evidence supporting mucosal healing and deep remission as important treatment goals for inflammatory bowel disease. Expert Rev Gastroenterol Hepatol 2016;1–13.

38. Hanauer SB, Kirsner JB. Treat the patient or treat the disease? Dig Dis 2012;30: 400–3.

39. Peyrin-Biroulet L, Sandborn W, Sands BE, et al. Selecting therapeutic targets in inflammatory bowel disease (STRIDE): determining therapeutic goals for treat-to-target. Am J Gastroenterol 2015;110:1324–38.

40. Zallot C, Peyrin-Biroulet L. Deep remission in inflammatory bowel disease: looking beyond symptoms. Curr Gastroenterol Rep 2013;15:315.
41. Carvalho PB, Rosa B, Cotter J. Mucosal healing in Crohn's disease - are we reaching as far as possible with capsule endoscopy? J Crohns Colitis 2014; 8(11):1566–7.
42. Cotter J, Dias de Castro F, Magalhaes J, et al. Validation of the Lewis score for the evaluation of small-bowel Crohn's disease activity. Endoscopy 2014;47(4): 330–5.
43. Efthymiou A, Viazis N, Mantzaris G, et al. Does clinical response correlate with mucosal healing in patients with Crohn's disease of the small bowel? A prospective, case-series study using wireless capsule endoscopy. Inflamm Bowel Dis 2008;14:1542–7.
44. Hall BJ, Holleran GE, Smith SM, et al. A prospective 12-week mucosal healing assessment of small bowel Crohn's disease as detected by capsule endoscopy. Eur J Gastroenterol Hepatol 2014;26:1253–9.
45. Hall B, Holleran G, Chin JL, et al. A prospective 52 week mucosal healing assessment of small bowel Crohn's disease as detected by capsule endoscopy. J Crohns Colitis 2014;8(12):1601–9.
46. Niv E, Fishman S, Kachman H, et al. Sequential capsule endoscopy of the small bowel for follow-up of patients with known Crohn's disease. J Crohns Colitis 2014; 8(12):1616–23.
47. Rutgeerts P, Geboes K, Vantrappen G, et al. Predictability of the postoperative course of Crohn's disease. Gastroenterology 1990;99:956–63.
48. Olaison G, Smedh K, Sjodahl R. Natural course of Crohn's disease after ileocolic resection: endoscopically visualised ileal ulcers preceding symptoms. Gut 1992; 33:331–5.
49. De Cruz P, Kamm MA, Hamilton AL, et al. Crohn's disease management after intestinal resection: a randomised trial. Lancet 2014;385(9976):1406–17.
50. Vaughn BP, Moss AC. Prevention of post-operative recurrence of Crohn's disease. World J Gastroenterol 2014;20:1147–54.
51. Bourreille A, Jarry M, D'Halluin PN, et al. Wireless capsule endoscopy versus ileocolonoscopy for the diagnosis of postoperative recurrence of Crohn's disease: a prospective study. Gut 2006;55:978–82.
52. Beltran VP, Nos P, Bastida G, et al. Evaluation of postsurgical recurrence in Crohn's disease: a new indication for capsule endoscopy? Gastrointest Endosc 2007;66:533–40.
53. Kopylov U, Rosenfeld G, Bressler B, et al. Clinical utility of fecal biomarkers for the diagnosis and management of inflammatory bowel disease. Inflamm Bowel Dis 2014;20(4):742–56.
54. Langhorst J, Elsenbruch S, Koelzer J, et al. Noninvasive markers in the assessment of intestinal inflammation in inflammatory bowel diseases: performance of fecal lactoferrin, calprotectin, and PMN-elastase, CRP, and clinical indices. Am J Gastroenterol 2008;103:162–9.
55. Kopylov U, Ben-Horin S, Seidman EG, et al. Video capsule endoscopy of the small bowel for monitoring of Crohn's disease. Inflamm Bowel Dis 2015;21: 2726–35.
56. Cave D, Legnani P, de Franchis R, et al. ICCE consensus for capsule retention. Endoscopy 2005;37:1065–7.
57. Cheifetz AS, Kornbluth AA, Legnani P, et al. The risk of retention of the capsule endoscope in patients with known or suspected Crohn's disease. Am J Gastroenterol 2006;101:2218–22.

58. Esaki M, Matsumoto T, Watanabe K, et al. Use of capsule endoscopy in patients with Crohn's disease in Japan: a multicenter survey. J Gastroenterol Hepatol 2014;29:96–101.

59. Nemeth A, Kopylov U, Koulaouzidis A, et al. Use of patency capsule in patients with established Crohn's disease. Endoscopy 2016;48:373–9.

60. Carter D, Lang A, Eliakim R. Endoscopy in inflammatory bowel disease. Minerva Gastroenterol Dietol 2013;59:273–84.

61. Li F, Gurudu SR, De Petris G, et al. Retention of the capsule endoscope: a single-center experience of 1000 capsule endoscopy procedures. Gastrointest Endosc 2008;68:174–80.

62. Hartmann D. Capsule endoscopy and Crohn's disease. Dig Dis 2011;29(Suppl 1):17–21.

63. Signorelli C, Rondonotti E, Villa F, et al. Use of the given patency system for the screening of patients at high risk for capsule retention. Dig Liver Dis 2006;38: 326–30.

64. Banerjee R, Bhargav P, Reddy P, et al. Safety and efficacy of the M2A patency capsule for diagnosis of critical intestinal patency: Results of a prospective clinical trial. J Gastroenterol Hepatol 2007;22:2060–3.

65. Caunedo-Alvarez A, Romero-Vazquez J, Herrerias-Gutierrez JM. Patency and Agile capsules. World J Gastroenterol 2008;14:5269–73.

66. Boivin ML, Lochs H, Voderholzer WA. Does passage of a patency capsule indicate small-bowel patency? A prospective clinical trial? Endoscopy 2005;37: 808–15.

67. Delvaux M, Ben Soussan E, Laurent V, et al. Clinical evaluation of the use of the M2A patency capsule system before a capsule endoscopy procedure, in patients with known or suspected intestinal stenosis. Endoscopy 2005;37:801–7.

68. Spada C, Shah SK, Riccioni ME, et al. Video capsule endoscopy in patients with known or suspected small bowel stricture previously tested with the dissolving patency capsule. J Clin Gastroenterol 2007;41:576–82.

69. Rozendorn N, Klang E, Lahat A, et al. Prediction of patency capsule retention in known Crohn's disease patients by using magnetic resonance imaging. Gastrointest Endosc 2016;83:182–7.

70. Kopylov U, NA, Cebrian A, et al. Symptomatic retention of the patency capsule – a multicenter real life case series Endoscopy international open. in press.

71. Eliakim R, Magro F. Imaging techniques in IBD and their role in follow-up and surveillance. Nat Rev Gastroenterol Hepatol 2014;11:722–36.

72. Goldberg HI, Caruthers SB Jr, Nelson JA, et al. Radiographic findings of the National Cooperative Crohn's Disease Study. Gastroenterology 1979;77:925–37.

73. Murphy SJ, Kornbluth A. Double balloon enteroscopy in Crohn's disease: where are we now and where should we go? Inflamm Bowel Dis 2011;17:485–90.

74. Pennazio M. Crohn's disease: diagnostic and therapeutic potential of modern small-bowel endoscopy. Gastrointest Endosc 2007;66:S91–3.

75. Wibmer AG, Kroesen AJ, Gröne J, et al. Comparison of strictureplasty and endoscopic balloon dilatation for stricturing Crohn's disease—review of the literature. Int J Colorectal Dis 2010;25:1149–57.

76. Greener T, Shapiro R, Klang E, et al. Clinical Outcomes of surgery versus endoscopic balloon dilation for stricturing Crohn's disease. Dis Colon Rectum 2015;58: 1151–7.

77. Hassan C, Zullo A, De Francesco V, et al. Systematic review: endoscopic dilatation in Crohn's disease. Aliment Pharmacol Ther 2007;26:1457–64.

78. Pennazio M. Capsule endoscopy: where are we after 6 years of clinical use? Dig Liver Dis 2006;38:867–78.
79. Grübel P, Choi Y, Schneider D, et al. Dig Dis Sci 2003;48:1360–5.
80. Benz C, Jakobs R, Riemann JF. Does the insertion depth in push enteroscopy depend on the working length of the enteroscope? Endoscopy 2002;34:543–5.
81. Benz C, Jakobs R, Riemann JF. Do we need the overtube for push-enteroscopy? Endoscopy 2001;33:658–61.
82. May A, Nachbar L, Schneider M, et al. Prospective Comparison of Push Enteroscopy and Push-and-Pull Enteroscopy in Patients with Suspected Small-Bowel Bleeding. Am J Gastroenterol 2006;101:2016–24.
83. Khashab MA, Lennon AM, Dunbar KB, et al. A comparative evaluation of single-balloon enteroscopy and spiral enteroscopy for patients with mid-gut disorders. Gastrointest Endosc 2010;72:766–72.
84. May A, Färber M, Aschmoneit I, et al. Prospective multicenter trial comparing push-and-pull enteroscopy with the single- and double-balloon techniques in patients with small-bowel disorders. Am J Gastroenterol 2010;105:575–81.
85. Heine GD, Hadithi M, Groenen MJ, et al. Double-balloon enteroscopy: indications, diagnostic yield, and complications in a series of 275 patients with suspected small-bowel disease. Endoscopy 2006;38:42–8.
86. Mensink P, Haringsma J, Kucharzik T, et al. Complications of double balloon enteroscopy: a multicenter survey. Endoscopy 2007;39:613–5.
87. Buscaglia J, Dunbar K, Okolo P, et al. The spiral enteroscopy training initiative: results of a prospective study evaluating the Discovery SB overtube device during small bowel enteroscopy (with video). Endoscopy 2009;41:194–9.
88. Chauhan SS, Manfredi MA, Abu Dayyeh BK, et al. Enteroscopy. Gastrointest Endosc 2015;82:975–90.

Role of Histologic Inflammation in the Natural History of Ulcerative Colitis

 CrossMark

Deepa T. Patil, MD[a],*, Alan C. Moss, MD, FACG, FEBG, AGAF, FRCPI[b],
Robert D. Odze, MD, FRCPC[c]

KEYWORDS

- Ulcerative colitis • Histology • Prognosis • Severity

KEY POINTS

- Several histologic grading systems exist to document the severity of ulcerative colitis (UC).
- These systems have not been validated for universal use in evaluating changes in histologic findings in response to therapy.
- Histologic features have been associated with clinical outcomes in patients with UC.

INTRODUCTION

Ulcerative colitis (UC) is a chronic, episodic inflammatory disorder of the colon that classically affects the rectum, with variable, but continuous, involvement of the proximal colon. The clinical management of UC primarily includes aminosalicylates, corticosteroids, purine antimetabolites, and tumor necrosis factor antagonists, either used sequentially or in combination.[1] The goal of medical therapy is to achieve clinical remission. In current clinical practice, disease activity is monitored by assessing patients' clinical symptoms and severity of colonic inflammation by colonoscopy. Consensus guidelines for clinical practice and trial end points recommend striving beyond resolution of clinical symptoms to achieve endoscopic mucosal healing. Endoscopic mucosal healing in inflammatory bowel disease (IBD) is defined by resolution of visible mucosal inflammation and ulceration. Several studies have shown that mucosal healing, as assessed by endoscopic examination, is associated with better long-term clinical outcomes compared with evaluation of clinical symptoms alone.[2–5]

Disclosure Statement: The authors have nothing to disclose.
[a] Cleveland Clinic, 9500 Euclid Av, L-25, Cleveland, OH 44195, USA; [b] Harvard Medical School, 330 Brookline Ave., Boston, MA 02215, USA; [c] Gastrointestinal Pathology, Brigham and Women's Hospital, Harvard Medical School, Boston, MA, USA
* Corresponding author.
E-mail address: patild@ccf.org

However, there is evidence to suggest that endoscopic findings do not necessarily correlate with histologic disease, especially after treatment.[6,7] Numerous scoring systems have been developed to measure the histologic features of UC and predict clinical outcome. The goal of this article is to (1) review the general pathologic features of UC, (2) review effects of medications on histology of UC, (3) discuss the pattern of histology in patients in clinical remission, and (4) address key histologic features predictive of relapse of disease or development of neoplasia.

PATHOLOGIC FEATURES OF ULCERATIVE COLITIS

Depending on the phase of disease and the degree of inflammatory activity, UC is categorized as *normal* (no histologic abnormalities) (**Fig. 1**), *chronic inactive* (**Fig. 2**), or *chronic active* (**Figs. 3** and **4**). Some patients may show activity but without features of chronicity (**Box 1**). Chronic colitis (regardless of presence or absence of activity) is defined by the presence of histologic features indicating chronic repeated tissue injury, such as crypt architectural distortion, crypt atrophy, diffuse mixed lamina propria inflammation, basal plasmacytosis, basal lymphoid aggregates, lamina propria fibrosis, pyloric gland metaplasia, and Paneth cell metaplasia, among others. Histologically, untreated UC involves the colon in a diffuse and continuous manner. It always involves the distal most portion of rectum (except in children in rare cases). UC characteristically involves the mucosa and occasionally the superficial submucosa in severe cases. The inflammatory infiltrate is typically composed of lymphocytes, plasma cells, and a variable amount of eosinophils and neutrophils depending on the severity of activity. The density of plasma cells is usually greatest in the basal region of the lamina propria (termed *basal plasmacytosis*). Basal lymphoid aggregates are also commonly present. A characteristic morphologic feature of UC is crypt architectural distortion. When distorted, crypts usually appear irregular, distended, branched, dilated, and/or foreshortened. It is considered a histologic hallmark of

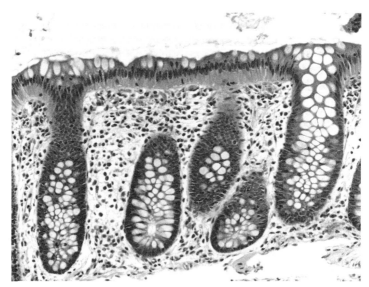

Fig. 1. Normal colon. The biopsy shows crypts that are arranged in a regular, test tube–like configuration. The lamina propria is composed of lymphocytes, plasma cells, and rare eosinophils. Hematoxylin-eosin, original magnification ×200.

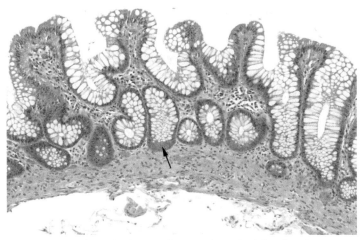

Fig. 2. Chronic inactive colitis. The biopsy obtained from the left colon shows crypt architectural distortion (irregular size and shape of the crypts) along with Paneth cell metaplasia (*arrow*). The lamina propria is slightly expanded by lymphocytes and plasma cells. There is no evidence of activity (neutrophils or eosinophils within the epithelium). Hematoxylin-eosin, original magnification ×100.

chronic injury. However, this feature is much more common in pretreatment, whereas in posttreatment the mucosa often normalizes completely without any evidence of crypt distortion. In a study that evaluated histologic changes following 5-aminosalicylic acid (5-ASA) treatment, crypt distortion was observed in 43% of cases.[8]

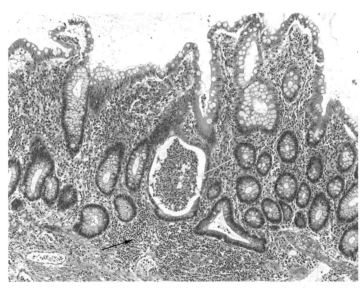

Fig. 3. Chronic active colitis with mild to moderate activity. The biopsy shows crypt architectural distortion along with expansion of the lamina propria by lymphoplasmacytic inflammatory cell infiltrate. Basal lymphoid aggregate is also present (*black arrow*). A large crypt abscess is also identified (*yellow arrow*). Hematoxylin-eosin, original magnification ×100.

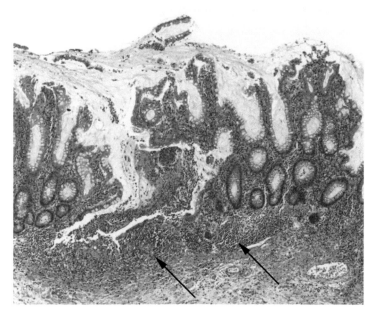

Fig. 4. Chronic active colitis with severe activity. The biopsy shows foci of neutrophilic epithelial injury along with erosion. In addition, there is prominent basal lymphoplasmacy-tosis (*arrows*) as well as crypt architectural distortion, all indicating chronic colitis with severe activity. Hematoxylin-eosin, original magnification ×40.

Box 1
Histologic features of activity and chronicity in ulcerative colitis

Common features of activity

- Increased eosinophils and neutrophils within the lamina propria
- Eosinophilic or neutrophilic infiltration within the crypt epithelium (cryptitis) with or without abscess formation (crypt abscesses)
- Surface erosion and/or ulceration
- Hemorrhage and edema within lamina propria
- Expansion of lamina propria by a mixed inflammatory cell infiltrate
- Regenerative epithelial changes, including mucin depletion

Common features of chronicity

- Crypt architectural distortion/atrophy
- Basal plasmacytosis
- Basal lymphoid aggregates
- Paneth cell metaplasia in left colon, Paneth cell hyperplasia in right colon
- Pyloric gland metaplasia
- Fibrosis
- Diffuse mixed lamina propria inflammation

The histologic features of active colitis vary depending on the severity of disease. In most active cases, a neutrophilic inflammatory cell infiltrate (either with or without eosinophils) may be present within the lamina propria and in the crypt epithelium (cryptitis). When neutrophils penetrate into the lumen of crypts and are associated with necrotic debris, it is termed *crypt abscess*. These abscesses are common in moderate to severe disease. Crypt abscesses may be focal or diffuse, depending on the severity of disease. Rupture of inflamed crypts can lead to the development of a granulomatous response to extravasated mucin. These crypt rupture–associated granulomas should be distinguished from granulomas in Crohn's disease.

HISTOLOGIC SCORING SYSTEMS TO ASSESS DISEASE ACTIVITY IN ULCERATIVE COLITIS

Truelove and Richards were the first to introduce a histologic scoring system that was applied to biopsy specimens from patients with UC.[9] Since then, there have been at least 18 histologic indices that have been proposed to measure to degree of inflammation in UC. Some of these include evaluating the degree of acute or chronic inflammation, inflammatory cell infiltrate within lamina propria and epithelium, architectural distortion, and integrity of colonic epithelium.[10] However, there is no universally accepted method of assessing activity in biopsies of patients with IBD. One commonly used method scores activity as inactive if there is no evidence of activity (defined as epithelial infiltration by neutrophils), mild if less than 50% of the mucosa shows evidence of activity, moderate if more than 50% shows these features, and severe if surface erosion or ulceration is present.[11] This method is the most commonly used method in clinical practice.

Review of the scoring systems used in clinical studies indicates that some systems use a stepwise method whereby the disease activity is divided into subjectively assessed grades, whereas others use a quantitative method by generating numerical scores that correspond to specific histologic features. Summarizing the strengths and limitations of all the 18 histologic scoring systems is beyond the scope of this review. The authors briefly discuss systems that have been commonly used in clinical studies and trials.

The Riley scoring system[12] uses a 4-point score (none, mild, moderate, and severe) to assess 6 histologic features: presence of an acute inflammatory cell infiltrate (neutrophils in the lamina propria), crypt abscesses, mucin depletion, surface epithelial integrity, chronic inflammatory cell infiltrate (round cells in the lamina propria), and crypt architectural irregularities. This scoring system was applied in a prospective study that was aimed at predicting recurrence in 82 outpatients with asymptomatic UC in endoscopic remission. This scoring system was later modified (Modified Riley Score)[13] to rank the degree of inflammation hierarchically and to exclude crypt architectural changes, which according to the investigators are not responsive to clinically relevant changes in inflammation. This system has never been validated but has been used in multiple randomized control trials.[10]

Geboes and colleagues[14] developed a scoring system that categorizes histologic changes as grade 0 (structural change only), grade 1 (chronic inflammation), grade 2 (a, lamina propria neutrophils; b, lamina propria eosinophils), grade 3 (neutrophils in the epithelium), grade 4 (crypt destruction), and grade 5 (erosions or ulcers) and generates a score from 0 to 5.4 that increases with disease severity or activity. The Geboes index has been applied to a few prospective clinical studies.[10,15] Although the Riley study did not address the interobserver and intraobserver variability among pathologists in scoring the histologic variables, the Geboes scoring system has been shown to be reproducible to some degree, whereby the investigators found moderate to good interobserver agreement among 3 pathologists (kappa 0.59–0.70).

Gramlich and colleagues[16] referred to activity as infiltration of neutrophils into the crypt epithelium. They classified activity as mild if there are rare neutrophils infiltrating the crypt epithelium, moderate if there are crypt abscesses, and severe if there are ulcers. In contrast to other systems, it does not incorporate neutrophils within the lamina propria as an indicator of activity and does not provide any clarity about scoring erosions.

Another index that was specifically developed to assess risk of neoplastic progression in UC is the Gupta index.[11] This system is the same that is used by pathologists in clinical practice, described earlier.

The Gramlich and Gupta indices grade activity by assessing neutrophil-mediated epithelial injury; the Geboes and Riley index also include crypt architectural changes, chronic inflammatory infiltrate within lamina propria, and eosinophils, providing a much more comprehensive assessment of histologic changes. More importantly, none of these scoring systems specifically assess basal plasmacytosis or provide thresholds for normal lamina propria inflammatory cells, especially mononuclear cells and eosinophils, the density of which is known to vary with anatomic location of the biopsy as well as geographic location of patients. Individuals who live in the southern United States and closer to the equator have more numbers of lamina propria eosinophils compared with the northern states.[17,18]

More recently, Mosli and colleagues[9] assessed the intraobserver and interobserver variability in applying the Geboes and Modified Riley Score using digital images.[10] Crypt architectural distortion, chronic inflammatory cell infiltrate, neutrophil-mediated epithelial injury, and erosions/ulcers had the highest intraclass correlation coefficient scores, whereas there was poor interobserver agreement in assessing lamina propria eosinophils and basal plasmacytosis.

EFFECT OF MEDICAL TREATMENT ON HISTOLOGY OF ULCERATIVE COLITIS

The first line of therapy for patients with UC usually includes aminosalicylates, corticosteroids, and immunomodulating agents (azathioprine or 6-mercaptopurine). However, a significant proportion of patients do not respond to these agents and, thus, either require additional therapy, such as intravenous cyclosporine, infliximab, adalimumab, or vedolizumab, or ultimately colectomy. In most studies that have evaluated the efficacy of these agents in the setting of randomized control trials, the end points of assessing outcome have included clinical symptoms and/or endoscopic appearance/healing. In some studies that have included histologic evaluation,[19–24] improvement was assessed in sigmoid colon or rectal biopsies using a grading system that includes no, mild, moderate, or severe activity. Thus, there is very limited information regarding the specific effects of individual therapeutic agents on the histology of UC. In general, in patients who have received medical therapy (oral or enema), mucosal histologic changes may vary considerably. Some or all portions of mucosa may heal completely and, as a result, show completely normal-appearing colonic mucosa histologically, without chronicity or activity. However, in many cases, endoscopically normal-appearing mucosa may show chronic inactive colitis, whereas others may show persistent active disease in the form of chronic active or only active features. Healing most often occurs in a segmental or patchy/uneven fashion.

In 1993, Odze and colleagues[23] prospectively evaluated 123 rectal mucosal biopsy specimens from 14 patients with pathologically confirmed UC treated with either 5-ASA or placebo enemas.[8] Overall, over the course of treatment, 29% of rectal biopsies from 64% of patients were histologically normal, showing no evidence of chronic or active disease. Furthermore, reversion to normal biopsies was more frequent in the 5-ASA-treated group indicating that prior treatment has a positive healing effect on the mucosa at the histologic level. Subsequent studies by Kleer and Appelman,[25] Bernstein and colleagues,[26] and Kim and colleagues[27] evaluated patchiness of disease and patterns of involvement in UC colorectal biopsy specimens over time. In these studies, 30% to 59% of patients, some of whom were treated with oral sulfasalazine or steroids (or both), showed either patchiness of disease or rectal sparing on follow-up surveillance biopsies, further supporting the idea that oral treatment often results in reversion of inflamed mucosa to one that is completely normal.

In a recent study by Tursi and colleagues,[27] a higher percentage of persistent histologic inflammation was found in patients with left-sided and distal colitis treated with infliximab.[28] On follow-up, histologic inflammation improved in patients with pancolitis compared with those with left-sided or distal colitis. Similarly, vedolizumab, an anti-integrin monoclonal antibody, has been reported to induce improvement in histologic grade in 50% of subjects with IBD treated in a small cohort.[29]

HISTOLOGY OF PATIENTS IN CLINICAL REMISSION

The European Crohn's and Colitis Organization[30] and the International Organization for the study of IBD (IOIBD)[31] define remission as complete resolution of symptoms and endoscopic mucosal healing. Endoscopic mucosal healing in UC is defined by resolution of visible mucosal inflammation and ulceration, often assessed by using the Mayo endoscopic scoring method.[32] Deep remission is a more recent concept in IBD management. It is currently defined as the combination of clinical remission and mucosal healing.[5,33] This concept has been relatively better characterized in Crohn's disease than UC.

Most patients with UC who are clinically asymptomatic eventually enter a resolving, or healing, phase of disease, characterized by decreasing activity (and symptoms) after an active colitis episode. This phase of disease is characterized morphologically by less activity and less crypt injury but higher levels of crypt regeneration and remodeling. Neutrophils, and other active components of crypt injury, decrease first followed later by a reduction in lamina propria lymphocytes and plasma cells. During this initial healing phase, there is often quite a lot of variability in the type and degree of mucosal inflammatory changes within biopsy fragments from different regions of the colon and even within individual fragments of mucosa itself. Thus, at any given point of time, endoscopic mucosal biopsies from patients with treated UC may show active colitis, chronic active colitis, chronic inactive colitis (with crypt architectural distortion), or completely normal mucosa on histologic examination. In fact, histologic inflammation was found in 54% of patients with UC who received maintenance therapy, and 37% had at least moderate inflammation based on histology scores.[34] Another study found that 99% of patients with IBD under deep remission with both infliximab and adalimumab had histologically inactive disease.[33] Unfortunately, there is little information on the exact temporal correlation between endoscopic healing and histologic healing. In a study by Moum and colleagues,[34] it was suggested that the discrepancy between endoscopic and histologic involvement in patients with UC increases with time.[35] In this study, histopathologic examination showed more extensive disease than endoscopic findings in 4% at diagnosis and in 28% at follow-up in 1 year, whereas endoscopic findings showed more extensive disease than histopathologic examination in 18% at diagnosis and 12% at follow-up.

HISTOLOGIC FEATURES PREDICTIVE OF CLINICAL OUTCOME

A recent initiative by the IOIBD noted that further studies are needed to confirm the prognostic value of histologic remission beyond, or independent of, that associated with endoscopic remission alone.[36] In this context, validated scoring systems for evaluation of histologic severity in clinical trials are desirable. The histologic abnormalities described earlier have been useful in describing the extent and severity of inflammation in patients with colitis but have not been used for prognostic purposes in practice. However, much emphasis has recently been placed on the importance of mucosal healing as an outcome for therapies in patients with IBD.[36,37] This importance is based on cumulative evidence that patients with normal/near-normal appearing colonic mucosa seem to have a lower risk of disease relapse, hospitalization, surgery, and cancer than those with moderate-severe UC.[3,7,38] Consequently, current and future clinical trials place a greater emphasis on objective outcomes, such as mucosal healing, in assessing novel therapies.[39] Evaluation of the severity of histologic inflammation as an end point for drug therapy has not been part of standard clinical practice, although persistent endoscopic and histologic inflammation in the absence of clinical symptoms is common.[6,34] Patients with quiescent UC but with histologic inflammation are difficult to identify, as endoscopic measures of inflammation have variable correlation with symptoms. A small prospective study, presented only in abstract form, reported only modest agreement between clinical, endoscopic, and histologic measures of remission, with complete agreement in just 58% of 91 patients (kappa 0.44) and 89% agreement between endoscopy and histology.[40] Although these studies emphasize macroscopic (endoscopic) mucosal healing, microscopic changes remain present in many patients whose mucosa appears normal endoscopically.[34] Because lamina propria expansion and crypt architecture distortion are integral to the pathogenic process in chronic UC, persistent histologic inflammation may have distinct prognostic implications for patients.[36]

HISTOLOGIC PREDICTORS OF DISEASE RECURRENCE

Riley and colleagues[11] first reported that histologic grade, but not endoscopic appearance, predicted clinical relapse in a cohort of 82 patients with UC in clinical and endoscopic remission.[12] In this study, the presence of crypt abscesses or a breached surface epithelium (presumably indicating surface erosion) had the greatest magnitude of risk of clinical relapse during 12 months of follow-up. Since then, several groups have evaluated the association between Geboes', Riley's, and Truelove and Richards' measures of histologic inflammation and clinical outcomes.[12,41,42] A prospective study of 108 patients by Zenlea and colleagues concluded that only histologic grade (Geboes score), and not endoscopic appearance, independently predicted the risk of clinical relapse over 12 months in patients in clinical remission at baseline.[15] A higher risk of relapse was noted in studies of patients with persistent active microscopic inflammation, when compared with patients with normal histology.[12,38,43] Histologic remission was also associated with a lower rate of hospitalization during a median 29-month follow-up in a small cohort.[32] Studies from both Hefti and colleagues[40] and Rubin and colleagues[41] reported that an increased level of histologic inflammation could predict both colectomy and hospitalization in patients with UC.[41,42] Regarding specific abnormalities, the presence of basal plasmacytosis, defined as a dense infiltration of plasma cells in the lower one-third of the mucosa on biopsy specimens, was noted to be an independent predictor of a shorter time to relapse (hazard ratio, 4.5) in patients with UC in clinical remission.[38] Bessissow and colleagues[7] confirmed this unique risk factor in a separate study.[7] Another study by Zezos and colleagues[43] found increased numbers of lamina propria eosinophils in patients with active UC. Severe eosinophilic infiltration was the most significant predictor of treatment failure in patients with active UC.[44]

HISTOLOGIC PREDICTORS OF COLORECTAL NEOPLASIA

Several studies have also specifically looked at the risk of colorectal neoplasia based on histologic findings. These studies have mostly used nonvalidated measures of histologic inflammation. An early case-control study by Rutter and colleagues[44] graded histologic inflammation based on the degree of epithelial neutrophil infiltration (0–4) and associated this grade with risk of colorectal neoplasia.[45] They reported that histology grade was independently associated with risk of colorectal neoplasia (odds ratio 4.7). Since then, other studies have come to similar conclusions, based on the relative presence of neutrophils in the epithelium.[43] Importantly, larger studies have controlled for other factors associated with risk of colorectal cancer (CRC), including macroscopic inflammation and medications. Rubin and colleagues[42] expanded the range of mononuclear cell infiltrate included but determined that only intraepithelial granulocytes with/without crypt abscesses contributed to the risk of colorectal cancer or dysplasia.[43] In another study by Gupta and colleagues,[10] severity of microscopic inflammation over time was found to be an independent risk factor for developing advanced colorectal neoplasia among patients with long-standing UC.[46] It should be noted that these were all retrospective studies from hospital-based cohorts, so subject to the associated biases of this methodology and selection. Whether reversal of these abnormalities reduces the cancer risk is unknown, although mesalamine seems to have a modest benefit in this regard.[47]

LIMITATIONS OF USING HISTOLOGIC REMISSION INDICES IN CLINICAL PRACTICE

Besides lack of a validated standard system and lack of a clear definition of histologic remission and its impact on clinical outcome of the disease, certain technical aspects of optimizing histologic assessment also need to be considered. These aspects include optimizing the minimum number of biopsies that need to be obtained, anatomic location of biopsies, timing of biopsies, and comparison of pretreatment and posttreatment biopsies, ensuring proper orientation to assess architectural changes, surface abnormalities, and basal plasmacytosis, evaluating superimposed infections, such as cytomegalovirus, and assessing interobserver and intraobserver reproducibility of histologic parameters that are used to generate histologic scores. Given the variability in histologic findings following treatment, it is advisable that regardless of the endoscopic appearance, biopsy samples should be obtained throughout the entire colon. Some investigators advocate a minimum of 2 biopsies from the right, transverse, descending, sigmoid colon, and rectum.[48]

SUMMARY

In summary, histologic assessment is certainly an important element in the clinical management of UC. It provides information that can be used to predict the course of disease, remission, future surgical procedures, and risk of neoplasia. However, before these indices can be used in routine clinical practice, they need to refined and further validated in larger clinical studies. Given the potential importance of histologic healing in long-term outcomes with UC, and the limitations of using symptoms alone to screen for underlying macroscopic or microscopic inflammation, identification of surrogate markers of histologic inflammation are needed for clinical use in the office and efficient trial design.

REFERENCES

1. Danese S, Fiocchi C. Ulcerative colitis. N Engl J Med 2011;365(18):1713–25.
2. Pineton de Chambrun G, Peyrin-Biroulet L, Lémann M, et al. Clinical implications of mucosal healing for the management of IBD. Nat Rev Gastroenterol Hepatol 2010;7(1):15–29.
3. Ardizzone S, Cassinotti A, Duca P, et al. Mucosal healing predicts late outcomes after the first course of corticosteroids for newly diagnosed ulcerative colitis. Clin Gastroenterol Hepatol 2011;9(6):483–9.e3.
4. Frøslie KF, Jahnsen J, Moum BA, et al, IBSEN Group. Mucosal healing in inflammatory bowel disease: results from a Norwegian population-based cohort. Gastroenterology 2007;133(2):412–22.
5. Colombel JF, Rutgeerts P, Reinisch W, et al. Early mucosal healing with infliximab is associated with improved long-term clinical outcomes in ulcerative colitis. Gastroenterology 2011;141(4):1194–201.
6. Baars JE, Nuij VJAA, Oldenburg B, et al. Majority of patients with inflammatory bowel disease in clinical remission have mucosal inflammation. Inflamm Bowel Dis 2012;18(9):1634–40.
7. Bessissow T, Lemmens B, Ferrante M, et al. Prognostic value of serologic and histologic markers on clinical relapse in ulcerative colitis patients with mucosal healing. Am J Gastroenterol 2012;107(11):1684–92.
8. Odze R, Antonioli D, Peppercorn M, et al. Effect of topical 5-aminosalicylic acid (5-ASA) therapy on rectal mucosal biopsy morphology in chronic ulcerative colitis. Am J Surg Pathol 1993 Sep;17(9):869–75.
9. Truelove SC. Treatment of ulcerative colitis with local hydrocortisone. Br Med J 1956;2(5004):1267–72.
10. Mosli MH, Feagan BG, Sandborn WJ, et al. Histologic evaluation of ulcerative colitis: a systematic review of disease activity indices. Inflamm Bowel Dis 2014; 20(3):564–75.
11. Gupta RB, Harpaz N, Itzkowitz S, et al. Histologic inflammation is a risk factor for progression to colorectal neoplasia in ulcerative colitis: a cohort study. Gastroenterology 2007;133(4):1099–105 [quiz: 1340–1].
12. Riley SA, Mani V, Goodman MJ, et al. Microscopic activity in ulcerative colitis: what does it mean? Gut 1991;32(2):174–8.
13. Feagan BG, Greenberg GR, Wild G, et al. Treatment of ulcerative colitis with a humanized antibody to the alpha4beta7 integrin. N Engl J Med 2005;352(24): 2499–507.
14. Geboes K, Riddell R, Ost A, et al. A reproducible grading scale for histological assessment of inflammation in ulcerative colitis. Gut 2000;47(3):404–9.
15. Zenlea T, Yee EU, Rosenberg L, et al. Histology grade is independently associated with relapse risk in patients with ulcerative colitis in clinical remission: a prospective Study. Am J Gastroenterol 2016;111(5):685–90.
16. Gramlich T, Petras RE. Pathology of inflammatory bowel disease. Semin Pediatr Surg 2007;16(3):154–63.
17. Hurrell JM, Genta RM, Melton SD. Histopathologic diagnosis of eosinophilic conditions in the gastrointestinal tract. Adv Anat Pathol 2011;18(5):335–48.
18. Pascal RR, Gramlich TL, Parker KM, et al. Geographic variations in eosinophil concentration in normal colonic mucosa. Mod Pathol 1997;10(4):363–5.

19. Kruis W, Kiudelis G, Rácz I, et al. Once daily versus three times daily mesalazine granules in active ulcerative colitis: a double-blind, double-dummy, randomised, non-inferiority trial. Gut 2009;58(2):233–40.
20. Kruis W, Bar-Meir S, Feher J, et al. The optimal dose of 5-aminosalicylic acid in active ulcerative colitis: a dose-finding study with newly developed mesalamine. Clin Gastroenterol Hepatol 2003;1(1):36–43.
21. Lee FI, Jewell DP, Mani V, et al. A randomised trial comparing mesalazine and prednisolone foam enemas in patients with acute distal ulcerative colitis. Gut 1996;38(2):229–33.
22. Green JRB, Mansfield JC, Gibson JA, et al. A double-blind comparison of balsalazide, 6.75 g daily, and sulfasalazine, 3 g daily, in patients with newly diagnosed or relapsed active ulcerative colitis. Aliment Pharmacol Ther 2002;16(1):61–8.
23. Malchow H, Gertz B. CLAFOAM Study group. A new mesalazine foam enema (Claversal Foam) compared with a standard liquid enema in patients with active distal ulcerative colitis. Aliment Pharmacol Ther 2002;16(3):415–23.
24. Rao SS, Dundas SA, Holdsworth CD, et al. Olsalazine or sulphasalazine in first attacks of ulcerative colitis? A double blind study. Gut 1989;30(5):675–9.
25. Kleer CG, Appelman HD. Ulcerative colitis: patterns of involvement in colorectal biopsies and changes with time. Am J Surg Pathol 1998;22(8):983–9.
26. Bernstein CN, Shanahan F, Anton PA, et al. Patchiness of mucosal inflammation in treated ulcerative colitis: a prospective study. Gastrointest Endosc 1995;42(3):232–7.
27. Kim B, Barnett JL, Kleer CG, et al. Endoscopic and histological patchiness in treated ulcerative colitis. Am J Gastroenterol 1999;94(11):3258–62.
28. Tursi A, Elisei W, Picchio M, et al. Histological inflammation in ulcerative colitis in deep remission under treatment with infliximab. Clin Res Hepatol Gastroenterol 2015;39(1):107–13.
29. Christensen B, Goeppinger S, Colman R, et al. Vedolizumab in the treatment of IBD: The University of Chicago experience. Am J Gastroenterol 2015;110(1):S–866.
30. Stange EF, Travis SPL, Vermeire S, et al. European evidence-based Consensus on the diagnosis and management of ulcerative colitis: Definitions and diagnosis. J Crohns Colitis 2008;2(1):1–23.
31. D'Haens G, Sandborn WJ, Feagan BG, et al. A review of activity indices and efficacy end points for clinical trials of medical therapy in adults with ulcerative colitis. Gastroenterology 2007;132(2):763–86.
32. Bryant RV, Burger DC, Delo J, et al. Beyond endoscopic mucosal healing in UC: histological remission better predicts corticosteroid use and hospitalisation over 6 years of follow-up. Gut 2016;65(3):408–14.
33. Molander P, Sipponen T, Kemppainen H, et al. Achievement of deep remission during scheduled maintenance therapy with TNFα-blocking agents in IBD. J Crohns Colitis 2013;7(9):730–5.
34. Rosenberg L, Nanda KS, Zenlea T, et al. Histologic markers of inflammation in patients with ulcerative colitis in clinical remission. Clin Gastroenterol Hepatol 2013;11(8):991–6.
35. Moum B, Vatn M, Ekbom A. Endoscopic and histological evaluation of extent of disease in ulcerative colitis: Differences increase from diagnosis, and until follow-up one year later. Gastroenterology 1997;112:A–1090.
36. Bryant RV, Winer S, Travis SPL, et al. Systematic review: histological remission in inflammatory bowel disease. Is "complete" remission the new treatment paradigm? An IOIBD initiative. J Crohns Colitis 2014;8(12):1582–97.

37. Bouguen G, Levesque BG, Pola S, et al. Endoscopic assessment and treating to target increase the likelihood of mucosal healing in patients with Crohn's disease. Clin Gastroenterol Hepatol 2014;12(6):978–85.

38. Bitton A, Peppercorn MA, Antonioli DA, et al. Clinical, biological, and histologic parameters as predictors of relapse in ulcerative colitis. Gastroenterology 2001;120(1):13–20.

39. Peyrin-Biroulet L, Bressenot A, Kampman W. Histologic remission: the ultimate therapeutic goal in ulcerative colitis? Clin Gastroenterol Hepatol 2014;12(6): 929–34.e2.

40. Thomas S, Von Herbay A, Walsh A. How much agreement is there between histological, endoscopic and clinical assessments of remission in ulcerative colitis? Gut 2009;58(S1):A101.

41. Hefti MM, Chessin DB, Harpaz NH, et al. Severity of inflammation as a predictor of colectomy in patients with chronic ulcerative colitis. Dis Colon Rectum 2009; 52(2):193–7.

42. Rubin DT, Bradette M, Gabalec L, et al. Ulcerative Colitis Remission Status After Induction With Mesalazine Predicts Maintenance Outcomes: the MOMENTUM Trial. J Crohns Colitis 2016;10(8):925–33.

43. Rubin DT, Huo D, Kinnucan JA, et al. Inflammation is an independent risk factor for colonic neoplasia in patients with ulcerative colitis: a case-control study. Clin Gastroenterol Hepatol 2013;11(12):1601–8.e1–4.

44. Zezos P, Patsiaoura K, Nakos A, et al. Severe eosinophilic infiltration in colonic biopsies predicts patients with ulcerative colitis not responding to medical therapy. Colorectal Dis 2014;16(12):O420–30.

45. Rutter M, Saunders B, Wilkinson K, et al. Severity of inflammation is a risk factor for colorectal neoplasia in ulcerative colitis. Gastroenterology 2004;126(2):451–9.

46. Gupta RB, Harpaz N, Itzkowitz S, et al. Histologic inflammation is a risk factor for progression to colorectal neoplasia in ulcerative colitis: a cohort study. Gastroenterology 2007;133(4):1099–105 [quiz: 1340–1].

47. O'Connor A, Moss AC. Current and emerging maintenance therapies for ulcerative colitis. Expert Rev Gastroenterol Hepatol 2014;8(4):359–68.

48. Marchal Bressenot A, Riddell RH, Boulagnon-Rombi C, et al. Review article: the histological assessment of disease activity in ulcerative colitis. Aliment Pharmacol Ther 2015;42(8):957–67.

Noninvasive Testing for Mucosal Inflammation in Inflammatory Bowel Disease

 CrossMark

Marisa Iborra, MD, PhD, Belén Beltrán, MD, PhD, Pilar Nos, MD, PhD*

KEYWORDS

- Biomarker • Inflammatory bowel disease • Crohn's disease • Ulcerative colitis
- Fecal calprotectin • C-reactive protein

KEY POINTS

- Fecal and serologic biomarkers have gained increasing attention by the physicians for the diagnosis and follow-up of inflammatory bowel disease (IBD).
- Biomarkers are rapid, inexpensive and noninvasive, and can be used in different stages of the disease with high sensitivity and specificity.
- Fecal markers such as calprotectin and test for C-reactive protein are used to assess disease activity, predict relapse, and monitor the treatment response.
- New noninvasive tests are being studied and the future years look promising for IBD.

Inflammatory bowel disease (IBD), Crohn's disease (CD) and ulcerative colitis (UC), is characterized by a relapsing and remitting course that cause a chronic inflammation of the gastrointestinal tract. The classic treatment goal has been focused on the control of clinical symptoms and clinical remission to guide treatment. However, it has been well-known that clinical symptoms are frequently inconsistent with endoscopic findings, especially in CD.[1] More recently, the goal of mucosal healing has emerged as the new treatment target to change the evolution of the disease.[2]

Colonoscopy is the gold standard technique for the diagnosis and assessment in IBD. Nevertheless, this procedure has several limitations. It is a technique that consumes longer time and is invasive; at the same time, it requires dietary restriction and the preparation of the colon, which is unpleasant for the patient. Currently, there are new noninvasive biomarkers to improve the detection of disease activity, prognosis prediction, and treatment adjustment. Those biomarkers can avoid IBD patients to be evaluated unnecessarily with invasive, expensive endoscopic examinations.

Gastroenterology Department, Department of Digestive Disease, Centro de Investigación Biomédica en Red de Enfermedades Hepáticas y Digestivas (CIBERehd), La Fe University and Polytechnic Hospital, Av. Fernando Abril Martorell, 106, Valencia 46026, Spain
* Corresponding author.
E-mail address: pilarnos@gmail.com

Gastrointest Endoscopy Clin N Am 26 (2016) 641–656
http://dx.doi.org/10.1016/j.giec.2016.06.005
1052-5157/16/$ – see front matter © 2016 Elsevier Inc. All rights reserved.

This article discusses the advances in serum markers and stool markers of inflammation and how they serve as a complement for the monitoring of the disease and the eluding some endoscopies. Finally, we review recent technical advances and new kinds of biomarkers.

SEROLOGIC MARKERS AND ANTIBODIES

Several serologic tests have been used in IBD clinics. The existence of antibodies to microbial antigens highlights the abnormal immune response produced in IBD patients. The most investigated ones are perinuclear antineutrophil cytoplasmic antibodies (pANCAs) and anti-*Saccharomyces cerevisiae* antibodies (ASCAs), which have been used to improve the diagnosis of IBD to distinguish CD from UC.[3] Whereas ASCA are generally found in CD patients (39%–76% in CD vs 5%–26% in UC), pANCA are more common among UC patients (20%–85% in UC vs 2%–28% in CD).[3,4] The specificity of these 2 combined markers tends to be higher than sensitivity, and for this reason, these markers are more useful in the differentiation of the IBD subtypes than in population screening.[4] Although ASCA and pANCA may be used to identify high-risk patients with complicated disease course,[5–8] a metaanalysis has demonstrated inconsistent results owing to the heterogeneity of different studies.[9] Finally, ASCA and pANCA have also been tested for their relationship with the response to therapy.[7] In this sense, pANCA may identify a CD subgroup with a poorer response to infliximab.[10,11] The combination of pANCA+/ASCA− could be predictive of nonresponse to infliximab in patients with refractory luminal CD.[12] Nevertheless, this serotype has been associated with early clinical response to infliximab in UC patients.[13]

The presence of other antibodies to microbial antigens as antibodies to outer membrane porin (anti-OmpC), flagellin (anti-Cbir1), *Pseudomonas flourescens*–associated sequence I-2 (anti-I2), and antibodies to flagellin A4-Fla2 and Fla-X in around 50% of CD patients supporting the role of altered microbial sensing in the pathogenesis of the disease.[6,14] New antiglycan antibodies, such as antilaminaribioside carbohydrate IgG, antichitobioside carbohydrate IgA, antisynthetic manobioside antibodies has been associated with complicated disease phenotype (stricturing or penetrating complications) and risk for surgery in CD patients.[7,8,15,16] Moreover, the expression of I-2 antibodies against a bacterial antigen of *Pseudomonas fluorescens* has been associated with highly clinical response to fecal diversion in CD patients (clinical response of 94% with I-2 positive vs 18% with I-2 negative).[17]

Although in clinical practice these serologic markers are not commonly used, their role in the management of IBD patients requires further investigation and prospective studies to verify its usefulness.

BLOOD MARKERS OF ACUTE PHASE RESPONSE

C-reactive protein (CRP) and the erythrocyte sedimentation rate (ESR) are the most commonly available and used blood markers. CRP is an acute phase protein with a short half-life (19 hours).[18,19] It is produced by the hepatocytes in response to an inflammatory trigger (cytokines as IL-6, tumor necrosis factor [TNF]-α and IL-1β) associated with active IBD. However, CRP is not specific marker for intestinal inflammation and the levels are also increased in infections, autoimmune disorders or malignancy.[6] The CRP levels in health is less than 1 mg/L, and during acute IBD levels can increase by 100-fold.[6,19] Considerable single heterogeneity exists in CRP generation. Elevations in CRP are more common in CD than in UC by the elevation of IL-6 and the transmural condition in CD.[20] A study showed that a 10% of active CD patients had low CRP (<10 mg/L) and those patients had a predominance of pure ileal disease, low body index and structuring behavior.[21] Up to 25% of CD patients with endoscopic activity show normal levels of CRP.[22] Moreover, gene polymorphisms and genetic determinants of CRP levels have also been reported as an explanation for differences in CRP levels.[23,24]

ESR is an indirect quantification of inflammation, by means of an increase in plasma viscosity owing to elaboration of acute phase response proteins.[25] This marker is not specific for intestinal inflammation and several factors as age, gender, anemia, polycythemia, or pregnancy can influence the ESR by reducing its accuracy and specificity in IBD.[26] The ESR has a long half-life; its resolution is slower in response to changes in inflammation and has a smaller degree of change. It is less appropriate to detect changes in disease activity, nevertheless it remains widely used as a biomarker of IBD activity.[6,14]

Other Laboratory Markers

Many proinflammatory cytokines, which are stimulated in the acute phase response as TNF-α, interferon-β, and IL-1β, IL-6, and IL-8, may also be elevated in serum of IBD patients.[27] Other potential serum markers comprise adenosine deaminase, soluble ST2 and tryptophan.[25] Currently, none of these molecules is used in routine practice, and their use is exclusively for basic science studies.

Cellular components of blood may also show inflammation. In contrast with infectious diarrhea, the platelet count may be elevated in active CD, whereas the platelet volume is low.[28,29] Platelets increase in IBD contributes to the high-coagulated status and the high risk of thrombosis. In active IBD, the white blood cell count may be elevated, but it is not specific, it may be influenced by corticotherapy.[6] Red blood cell distribution has showed to be a good predictor of disease activity in CD patients without anemia.[30]

Serum albumin may be low, but it is also affected by nutritional status.[6] These changes may alarm the clinicians about ongoing inflammation.

URINE MARKERS

Several urine markers have been studied as potential predictors of activity in IBD.[25] The urinary excretion of urine isoprostaglandin F2α type III and leukotriene E have been correlated with clinical relapse and inflammation in CD patients.[31,32] Recently, prostaglandin E-major urinary metabolite has demonstrated better sensitivity for reflecting UC activity than CRP level.[33] Urine neopterin (a product of human monocytes/macrophages stimulated by interferon-γ) has been correlated with clinical activity of CD[34]; however, other studies have not found any changes.[35] The quantification of urinary metabolites could be an interesting noninvasive biomarker for the assessment of IBD activity. However, more studies are necessary to validate these results.

FECAL MARKERS

Stool markers are specific to the gastrointestinal tract, noninvasive, and inexpensive. For this reason, they have emerged as new diagnostic tools to detect mucosal inflammation. Fecal markers comprise a heterogeneous group of biological substances that are released by the inflamed mucosa.[25,36] The characteristics of those markers are laid out in **Table 1**.

Quantitative fecal excretion of indium 111-labeled leukocytes is considered the gold standard fecal marker of assessing disease activity in CD, specific for bowel inflammation.[37] However, it is not recommended in clinical practice owing to high cost, exposure to radiation, and discomfort because 4 days are necessary for fecal collection.

Table 1
Characteristics of the stools biomarkers in IBD: Pros and cons

Positive Attributes	Negative Attributes
Good acceptance and noninvasive	Patient's disinclination to collect stools
Inexpensive	Lack of specify in IBD
Reproducible (repetition of the text with the same process over time)	Intraindividual variability of fecal markers (day-to-day variation)
Rapid results (accelerate the decisions)	None have full validation for each scenario
Standardized	Lack of established cutoff levels
Predictive value for disease relapse, response to therapy, mucosal healing	Depend on physiologic factors (age, comorbidity)

Abbreviation: IBD, inflammatory bowel disease.

The fecal level of α1-antitrypsin (a protease inhibitor) is a reliable marker for intestinal protein loss and reflects clinical activity in CD. It is not accepted because it is not usually accessible and affordable.[14,38] Fecal excretion of α2-macroglobulin (a serum antiproteinase) has a positive correlation with activity in CD.[39] Similarly, fecal neopterin concentration is increased in patients with clinically active CD and UC patients.[35]

There are some neutrophil-derived proteins as lysozyme, myeloperoxidase, calprotectin, lactoferrin, and polymorphonuclear neutrophil elastase that are generally elevated in the feces of IBD patients and they are good indicators of disease activity.[14,40]

Fecal Calprotectin

Undoubtedly, the incorporation into routine of fecal calprotectin (FC) as a noninvasive, "gold standard" marker of intestinal inflammation has been a high advance in the management of IBD patients. The molecular pattern proteins S100A8/S100A9, which are damage-associated, collectively called calprotectin and S100A12, are also steady in stool, and are increased in active IBD. Calprotectin is a 36-kDa protein that mixes zinc and calcium and inhibits metalloproteinases. It has antimicrobial effects and induces apoptosis in cell cultures.[41] It is resistant to bacterial degradation in the gut and steady in feces, up to 7 days at room temperature. Its quantification in stool is by enzyme-linked immunosorbent assays. Calprotectin makes up 60% of granulocyte cytosolic protein, and is directly proportional with neutrophil migration toward the intestinal tract, making it a sensitive marker of inflammation.[6,14,36] FC can be produced by monocytes and possibly epithelial cells and is remarkably elevated in several conditions, including neoplasia, polyps, other inflammatory colitis (nonsteroidal antiinflammatory enteropathy, microscopic colitis, or allergic colitis), advancing age, celiac disease, and infections.[6,19,42] FC has shown to be able to identify patients with symptoms of IBD who should be further investigated for a possible IBD diagnosis and to monitor disease activity or to evaluate the response to therapy; in addition, it can predict a relapse and postoperative recurrence and has a good correlation with endoscopic and histologic activity. However, there are not any well-established cutoff levels because they vary according to the patient's condition.[43,44]

Fecal Lactoferrin

Lactoferrin is an iron-binding glycoprotein found in neutrophil granules with antimicrobial properties and is activated in acute inflammation.[6,40] It is steady for 5 days, resistant to freeze–thaw cycles and degradation; moreover, it is also measured by enzyme-linked immunosorbent assays, easing its use as a laboratory test. Contrasting with calprotectin, lactoferrin is specific to neutrophils.[6,40] A large number of studies included in a review have assessed the usefulness of fecal lactoferrin by reflecting endoscopic and histologic severity in IBD.[45] However, the results are inconsistent and it is necessary to validate the cutoffs.

Fecal S100A12

S100A12 is similar to calprotectin in its calcium-binding properties and it has high sensitivity and specificity (86% and 96%, respectively). In addition, it is easy to collect and detect, steady for 7 days at room temperature, inexpensive, and has good compliance.[25,40] This protein activates the nuclear factor-κB pathway and increases cytokine release. Although S1000A12 is also detectable in serum, the fecal essay is more sensitive and specific for IBD.[6,40] Several studies in pediatric and adult IBD patients have demonstrated its correlation with disease activity, response of treatment, mucosal healing, and disease relapse.[40]

Fecal Myeloperoxidase

Myeloperoxidase, an enzyme that works in the oxygen-dependent killing microorganisms, is released from the primary granules of neutrophils during acute inflammation.[14] The concentration of this enzyme is also proportional to the number of neutrophils within that region. Myeloperoxidase might be used as a surrogate marker for the determination of outcomes of successful treatment for IBD patients,[46] but it has not a good correlation with the severity of the endoscopic inflammation.[47] Later, fecal myeloperoxidase levels have been related to histologic indices of UC patients.[48] Further investigations are necessary to identify the clinical role of fecal myeloperoxidase in IBD.

Rectal Nitric Oxide

In response to acute proinflammatory cytokines, leukocytes and epithelial cells express inducible nitric oxide (NO) synthase, which leads to the production and accumulation of significant quantities of NO. The levels of NO, an endogenously produced gas, have been explored in serum,[49] exhaled[50] directly in the intestinal lumen (NO gas) in IBD patients.[51] According to this, the level of rectal NO has been correlated with the disease activity and the quantity of loose stools in IBD patients and great decrease in response to antiinflammatory treatment.[52,53] Moreover, low rectal NO levels are predictive of a poor clinical response to steroid treatment.[54]

Other fecal biomarkers are being investigated to be used in IBD patients. Although promise exist, these alternatives have shown less consistent results, lower correlation to disease activity, and overlap among patients with active and inactive disease.[55,56] These include lysozyme, leukocyte esterase, elastase, TNF-α, IL-1B, IL-4, IL-10, α1-antitrypsin, and α-2-macroglobulin.[25,32,57] M2-pyruvate kinase may be the most promising of these developing fecal biomarkers.[58]

THE CLINICAL USEFULNESS OF THE CURRENT BIOMARKERS IN INFLAMMATORY BOWEL DISEASE

Currently, biomarkers more widely used by physicians to monitor IBD patients are FC and CRP. The role of these tools in clinical practice is avoiding uncomfortable colonoscopies. These markers are able to select symptomatic patients for diagnosis of IBD, monitor response for treatment and mucosal healing, predict the relapse and the recurrence and select the IBD patients for endoscopy.[59] The properties and cutoff points of FC vary according to the type and location of disease, the disease context and the patient's age. Next, we explain the value of these tools in clinically relevant subgroups of patients. **Table 2** summarizes the cutoffs for FC suggested in each situation.

Usefulness in the Diagnosis of Inflammatory Bowel Disease

Gastroenterologist help many patients with nonspecific abdominal pain or diarrhea present in organic or functional disorders. The usefulness of the biomarkers in this context is to screen patients who would benefit from invasive and expensive techniques like colonoscopy or radiographs. A metaanalysis of studies of diagnostic accuracy demonstrated that FC can distinguish IBD from irritable bowel syndrome in adults between with a sensitivity of 93% and specificity of 96%.[66] In studies of children and teenagers, the sensitivity was similar to adults (92%); however, the specificity was lower (76%), probably because healthy children up to 9 years old had higher levels of FC.[66] This study showed FC is a useful screening tool for the investigation of suspected IBD and reduces the number of unnecessary endoscopic procedures. A recent systematic review and metaanalysis have revealed CRP and FC of 0.5 mg/dL or less or 40 μg/g or less, respectively, exclude IBD in patients with symptoms with a 99% probability.[67] The cutoff values of these studies range from 24 to 150 μg/g of stool.[25]

The Role of Biomarkers to Evaluate Disease Activity

Currently, it is known endoscopic disease activity is better correlated with biomarkers than with indices of clinical disease activity. A recent review with 28 studies showed the capacity of FC to determine endoscopic disease activity in IBD patients.[45] In CD patients the correlation between the CD Endoscopic Index Severity (CDEIS) and FC is considerably better than its correlation with CD Activity Index.[60] A value of 272 μg/g has demonstrated to be optimal distinguishing endoscopic remission (CDEIS <3).[62] Another study showed levels of 250 μg/g or less predicted endoscopic remission (CDEIS ≤3) with 94.1% sensitivity and 62.2% specificity.[60] A cutoff value of

Table 2
The usefulness of fecal calprotectin in the management of IBD patients

Study	No. of Patients	Disease	Cutoff Value (μg/g)	Sensitivity (%)	Specificity (%)
Correlation with endoscopic scores					
D'Haens et al,[60] 2012	126	CD	CDEIS <3: 250	94.1	62.2
		UC	Mayo >0: >250	71	100
Predicting clinical relapse					
Garcia-Sanchez et al,[61] 2010	69	UC	>120	80	60
	66	CD	>200		
Predicting postoperative recurrence					
Lobaton et al,[62] 2013	29	CD	203	75	72
Boschetti et al,[63] 2015	86	CD	100	95	54
Wright et al,[64] 2015	135	CD	100	89	58
Detection of pouchitis					
Yamamoto et al,[65] 2015	60	UC	56	100	84

Abbreviations: CD, Crohn's disease; CDEIS, CD Endoscopic Index Severity; IBD, inflammatory bowel disease; UC, ulcerative colitis.

250 μg/g indicated the presence of large ulcers in CD (sensitivity of 60.4% and specificity of 79.5%).[60] Moreover, FC has demonstrated improved usefulness for activity monitoring that other blood biomarkers and the clinical activity index (CRP, blood leukocytes, and CD Activity Index). It was the only marker that significantly discriminated inactive endoscopic disease from mild activity (104 ± 138 vs 231 ± 244 μg/g; $P<.001$), mild from moderate activity (231 ± 244 vs 395 ± 256 μg/g; $P = .008$), and moderate from high activity (395 ± 256 vs 718 ± 320 μg/g; $P<.001$).[68] However, the correlation between the FC levels and endoscopic activity seems better when the disease has ileocolonic or colonic involvement than when it is a pure ileal location.[62]

It seems FC levels show better correlation with endoscopically and histologically disease activity in UC than in CD.[69] In UC, an FC of greater than 250 μg/g presents a high sensitivity and specificity (71% and 100.0%, respectively) for active mucosal disease activity (Mayo Score >0). FC levels significantly correlates with symptom scores in UC ($r = 0.561$; $P<.001$), but not in CD.[60] Similar to CD, endoscopic disease activity correlates better with FC than other blood biomarkers and the clinical activity index (CRP, platelets, blood leukocytes, hemoglobin, and Lichtiger index).[70] FC is the only marker that can be discriminated among different grades of endoscopic activity (grade 0, 16 [10–30] μg/g; grade 1, 35 [25–48] μg/g; grade 2, 102 [44–159] μg/g; grade 3, 235 [176–319] μg/g; grade 4, 611 [406–868] μg/g; $P<.001$ for discriminating the different grades). A cutoff of 57 μg/g has got high sensitivity (91%) and specificity (90%) to detect endoscopically active disease (modified Baron Index ≥2).[70] Notably, histologic features of inflammation can be identified reliably based on their fecal level of calprotectin.[71] Patients with active histologic inflammation have got a significantly higher average level of FC than those without active histologic inflammation (278 vs 68 μg/g; $P = .002$).[71] Moreover, a recent study has demonstrated FC levels have got a good correlation with the degree of disease activity according to magnetic resonance enterography and with surgical pathology damage in ileal CD (Chiorean's score).[72] A cutoff value of 166.5 μg/g is predictive for a diagnosis of inflammation. No relationship is found for CRP.[72] In the same way, a good association between FC and small bowel inflammation score in capsule endoscopy (Lewis score) has been shown. A cutoff value of 76 μg/g is useful to determine appreciable visual inflammation in small bowel with a sensitivity of 59% and a specify of 41%.[73]

CRP is often increased in active transmural CD more than mild to moderate UC, responses based on extent of disease (less elevated in proctocolitis and left colitis and isolated small bowel CD) and it is a predictor of surgery in subgroups of patients with either UC or CD.[74] CRP elevations (>0.8 mg/dL) are associated with clinical disease activity and endoscopic inflammation in both CD and UC, and with severe active histologic inflammation only in CD patients.[75] Several studies have described a good correlation between CRP and activity endoscopy.[19] In CD patients on anti-TNF therapy, the CDEIS correlates better with CRP than with clinical indices (CD Activity Index and Harvey); however, CRP is not demonstrated to be reliable to identify endoscopic remission.[76]

The Role of Biomarkers to Prediction of Relapse

CF is able to detect subclinical mucosal inflammation and identify patients with risk of relapse. Different studies have demonstrated elevated CF in patients with clinical remission is associated with an increase of risk of relapse.[77,78] For example, an FC concentration greater than 150 μg/g showed a 2-fold and 14-fold increase in the relapse risk, respectively, in those patients with CD and UC in clinical remission.[77] A Spanish study demonstrated that FC concentration was higher among the patients with relapse than in those that remained in clinical remission (444 µg/g [95% CI, 34–983] vs 112 µg/g [95% CI, 22–996]; $P<.01$).[61] Finally, an FC of greater than 200 µg/g in CD and greater than 120 µg/g in UC were associated with a 4-fold and 6-fold increase in the probability of disease activity outbreak respectively.[61] Nevertheless, FC seems to be more useful in predicting relapse in UC and CD with colon involvement compared with isolated ileal CD, as mentioned.[61,78]

Finally, FC has demonstrated to be a good predictor of relapse in IBD patients under maintenance anti-TNFα therapy. In patients treated with infliximab, high levels of FC during maintenance therapy predict relapse within the following 2 months (332 ± 168 vs 110 ± 163 µg/g in relapsing and nonrelapsing disease, respectively). An FC of greater than 160 µg/g is predictive of relapse. In contrast, low FC levels are associated with a good response to treatment and long-term remission.[79] Similarly, patients on adalimumab maintenance therapy with low FC levels have got less probability of relapse than those with high FC levels (45 vs 625 µg/g). Small FC levels exclude relapse within at least 4 months after testing. The cutoff value to predict relapse is 204 µg/g.[80]

Similarly, high CRP levels (>15 mg/L) have been correlated with high severity clinical relapse in CD patients.[57] In quiescent CD, a higher CRP (>10 mg/L), fertilizing disease behavior, and disease confined to the colon are independent predictors of relapse.[81]

The Role of Biomarkers in the Evaluation of the Response to Treatment

Several studies have demonstrated the usefulness of the biomarkers determining the efficacy of treatment accurately and noninvasively. In clinical practice, the normalization of FC levels (<50 µg/g) in IBD patients after medical treatment is a marker that predicts mucosal healing.[46] Greater changes in FC after initiation of new therapy in active disease are correlated with better treatment response.[25] It has suggested for deescalation of any drug or cessation of corticosteroids or mesalamine, a confirmation of biological remission with FC and CRP could be enough.[69]

In UC patients in clinical remission but with an FC of greater than 50 µg/g, the intensification of mesalamine shows a significant decrease of FC level.[82] Kolho and colleagues[83] analyzed the ability of FC to reflect the response to glucocorticoid therapy. In acute UC, the levels of FC are high in patients that require colectomy, but not in corticosteroid and infliximab nonresponders.[55] A decrease of FC concentration in week 2 in UC patients undergoing induction infliximab therapy have been correlated with endoscopic remission in week 10.[84]

The pivotal studies such as CHARM,[56] ACCENT 1,[58] and SONIC[85] have evaluated the association between the response to treatment with anti-TNF antibodies and the decrease in CRP levels. A high stool frequency as well as a high CRP and low serum albumin are related to treatment failure in UC patients.[86] A high CRP level during relapse (>15 mg/L) has shown a better response to infliximab therapy and more severe clinical course in CD patients.[57] Magro and colleagues[87] demonstrate that baseline CRP values are higher in primary non response to infliximab patients when they are compared with those with sustained response (26.2 vs 9.6 mg/L; $P = .015$). Moreover, in this study, lower CRP levels at week 14 (<3 mg/L) are associated with sustained response (78% vs 57% achieved clinical response; $P = .053$).[87] According to this, the quick normalization of CRP levels correlates with sustained long-term response to infliximab (CRP <3 mg/L at week 4)[88,89] and adalimumab (CRP <10 mg/L at week 12).[90] In contrast, elevated CRP (>0.5 mg/dL) may be an indicator of low infliximab levels (<1 µg/mL) and, in consequence, it could predict loss of response and clinical relapse.[91]

The Role of Biomarkers to Predict Postoperative Recurrence

Surgery in CD is frequent, 80% of patients during their lifetime will need surgery and 70% of these patients will require second intestinal resection. Postoperative recurrence is common and clinical symptoms do not reflect recurrent endoscopic inflammation exactly. Treatment should be personalized and based on the risk of recurrence. Rapid detection of postoperative recurrence and subsequent quickly intervention will prevent new surgeries. Today, repetitive ileocolonoscopy is the gold standard to monitor the recurrence but it has many inconveniences. It is desirable to develop a good strategy by using biomarkers to determinate early postoperative recurrence.

FC usually returns to the normal level within 2 months of the surgery,[92] and its increase is associated with recurrence.[69] It has suggested a cutoff for FC of greater than 200 µg/mL is capable of identifying endoscopic recurrence at 1 year after surgery with 63% and 75% of sensitivity and specificity respectively.[93] Another study demonstrated that patients without significant recurrence (Rutgeerts score i0-1) had fewer CF levels than those with postoperative recurrence (Rutgeerts score 2-4; 98 µg/g [30–306] vs 234.5 µg/g [100–612], respectively).[62] The cutoff of value was 203 µg/g.[62] The POCER study (Post-Operative Crohn's Endoscopic Recurrence) explored the best strategy to prevent recurrence (defined as Rutgeerts $\geq$2) in postoperative CD patients.[94] Whereas FC levels of greater than 100 µg/g indicated endoscopic recurrence,[64] CRP did not correlate with disease recurrence.[94]

Few studies have evaluated the role of CRP in the prediction of postoperative CD recurrence and the data are not consistent. Although Regueiro and colleagues[95] did not find a correlation between CRP and endoscopic scores, Sorrentino and colleagues[96] showed a significant correlation between the procedures; nonetheless, the sample size in this study was small. A recent study with 86 CD patients found that patients in endoscopic remission had a lower CRP value than patients with recurrence (3 $\pm$ 0.7 vs 8.5 $\pm$ 1.4 mg/L; P = .0014).[63] However, there are not enough data supporting the use of CRP to determine postoperative recurrence.

FC seems better surrogate marker of endoscopy activity in recurrent CD than other clinical and serologic markers like CRP. The overall accuracy seems greater for FC (defined as >100 µg/g) than for hsCRP (defined as 1 mg/L; 77% vs 53%, respectively).[63] FC values of 100 µg/g or less strongly suggest recurrent disease and no need for further endoscopic procedures.

The Role of Biomarkers to Monitored Ileo–pouch–anal Anastomosis

The role of FC for early detection of pouchitis in patients with UC who have undergone proctocolectomy with ileo–pouch–anal anastomosis is highlighted. FC has been shown to distinguish reliably between inflamed and noninflamed pouches and correlate with the severity of pouchitis.[97,98] A recently prospective study has demonstrated that FC and lactoferrin levels are elevated 2 months before the diagnosis of pouchitis.[65] Patients with pouchitis after restorative proctocolectomy for UC have higher levels of FC than those without pouchitis. A cutoff value of 56 µg/g for FC has shown a sensitivity of 100% and a specificity of 84% to predict pouchitis, whereas a cutoff value of 50 µg/g for lactoferrin has reached a sensitivity of 90% and a specificity of 86%.[65] These fecal biomarkers can be useful for the early diagnosis of pouchitis and the detection of patients for colonoscopy assessment and therapeutic adjustment.

INVESTIGATION OF FUTURE APPROACHES

The investigation and testing of new IBD biomarkers is an area of active research. There are recent advances with new technologies and platforms capable of measuring thousands biospecimens simultaneously. This technology can be used to identify several markers including differences in gene expression, proteomics and metabolomics profiles, which suppose a significant advance in the management and knowledge of IBD.[6,25]

In addition to the first genome-wide association studies using single nucleotide polymorphisms, there are advances in the genetic investigations including pharmacogenetics studies and genetic testing for diagnosis and prognosis of IBD.[99] Recently, studies have focused on microRNA, small, noncoding RNA species that regulate gene expression. The role of microRNAs is yet to be understood, but it seems to be useful for peripheral blood and tissue biomarkers in IBD patients, with future clinical applications such as diagnostic and therapeutic targets, as well as future therapies.[100–102]

Proteomic studies have identified protein profiles in tissue, serum, or stools. Proteomic tools could be used for the diagnosis and prognosis of IBD, identifying active disease and predicting treatment response. The investigations suggest promising proteomic biomarkers like novel biomarkers and future targets that can help in the insight of the pathogenesis of the disease.[103]

The analysis of metabolic profile in IBD has emerged like tools for the diagnosis, potential biomarkers, and insight into the pathogenia of IBD.[25] Urine, serum, feces and colon tissue have been evaluated with promising results.[6] More recently, exhaled breath analysis of volatile organic compounds has emerged like a promising approach and noninvasive diagnostic tool for the diagnosis and assessment of IBD.[104,105]

REFERENCES

1. Cellier C, Sahmoud T, Froguel E, et al. Correlations between clinical activity, endoscopic severity, and biological parameters in colonic or ileocolonic Crohn's disease. A prospective multicentre study of 121 cases. The Groupe d'Etudes Therapeutiques des Affections Inflammatoires Digestives. Gut 1994;35(2): 231–5.
2. Papi C, Fasci-Spurio F, Rogai F, et al. Mucosal healing in inflammatory bowel disease: treatment efficacy and predictive factors. Dig Liver Dis 2013;45(12): 978–85.
3. Peyrin-Biroulet L, Standaert-Vitse A, Branche J, et al. IBD serological panels: facts and perspectives. Inflamm Bowel Dis 2007;13(12):1561–6.
4. Mokrowiecka A, Daniel P, Slomka M, et al. Clinical utility of serological markers in inflammatory bowel disease. Hepatogastroenterology 2009;56(89):162–6.
5. Russell RK, Ip B, Aldhous MC, et al. Anti-Saccharomyces cerevisiae antibodies status is associated with oral involvement and disease severity in Crohn disease. J Pediatr Gastroenterol Nutr 2009;48(2):161–7.
6. Iskandar HN, Ciorba MA. Biomarkers in inflammatory bowel disease: current practices and recent advances. Transl Res 2012;159(4):313–25.
7. Lewis JD. The utility of biomarkers in the diagnosis and therapy of inflammatory bowel disease. Gastroenterology 2011;140(6):1817–26.e2.
8. Mow WS, Vasiliauskas EA, Lin YC, et al. Association of antibody responses to microbial antigens and complications of small bowel Crohn's disease. Gastroenterology 2004;126(2):414–24.
9. Reese GE, Constantinides VA, Simillis C, et al. Diagnostic precision of anti-Saccharomyces cerevisiae antibodies and perinuclear antineutrophil cytoplasmic antibodies in inflammatory bowel disease. Am J Gastroenterol 2006; 101(10):2410–22.

10. Taylor KD, Plevy SE, Yang H, et al. ANCA pattern and LTA haplotype relationship to clinical responses to anti-TNF antibody treatment in Crohn's disease. Gastroenterology 2001;120(6):1347–55.

11. Dubinsky MC, Mei L, Friedman M, et al. Genome wide association (GWA) predictors of anti-TNFalpha therapeutic responsiveness in pediatric inflammatory bowel disease. Inflamm Bowel Dis 2010;16(8):1357–66.

12. Esters N, Vermeire S, Joossens S, et al. Serological markers for prediction of response to anti-tumor necrosis factor treatment in Crohn's disease. Am J Gastroenterol 2002;97(6):1458–62.

13. Ferrante M, Vermeire S, Katsanos KH, et al. Predictors of early response to infliximab in patients with ulcerative colitis. Inflamm Bowel Dis 2007;13(2):123–8.

14. Turkay C, Kasapoglu B. Noninvasive methods in evaluation of inflammatory bowel disease: where do we stand now? An update. Clinics (Sao Paulo) 2010;65(2):221–31.

15. Ferrante M, Henckaerts L, Joossens M, et al. New serological markers in inflammatory bowel disease are associated with complicated disease behaviour. Gut 2007;56(10):1394–403.

16. Papp M, Altorjay I, Dotan N, et al. New serological markers for inflammatory bowel disease are associated with earlier age at onset, complicated disease behavior, risk for surgery, and NOD2/CARD15 genotype in a Hungarian IBD cohort. Am J Gastroenterol 2008;103(3):665–81.

17. Spivak J, Landers CJ, Vasiliauskas EA, et al. Antibodies to I2 predict clinical response to fecal diversion in Crohn's disease. Inflamm Bowel Dis 2006; 12(12):1122–30.

18. Pepys MB, Hirschfield GM. C-reactive protein: a critical update. J Clin Invest 2003;111(12):1805–12.

19. Chang S, Malter L, Hudesman D. Disease monitoring in inflammatory bowel disease. World J Gastroenterol 2015;21(40):11246–59.

20. Gross V, Andus T, Caesar I, et al. Evidence for continuous stimulation of interleukin-6 production in Crohn's disease. Gastroenterology 1992;102(2): 514–9.

21. Florin TH, Paterson EW, Fowler EV, et al. Clinically active Crohn's disease in the presence of a low C-reactive protein. Scand J Gastroenterol 2006;41(3):306–11.

22. Vermeire S, Van Assche G, Rutgeerts P. C-reactive protein as a marker for inflammatory bowel disease. Inflamm Bowel Dis 2004;10(5):661–5.

23. Carlson CS, Aldred SF, Lee PK, et al. Polymorphisms within the C-reactive protein (CRP) promoter region are associated with plasma CRP levels. Am J Hum Genet 2005;77(1):64–77.

24. Danik JS, Ridker PM. Genetic determinants of C-reactive protein. Curr Atheroscler Rep 2007;9(3):195–203.

25. Sands BE. Biomarkers of Inflammation in Inflammatory Bowel Disease. Gastroenterology 2015;149(5):1275–85.e2.

26. Mendoza JL, Abreu MT. Biological markers in inflammatory bowel disease: practical consideration for clinicians. Gastroenterol Clin Biol 2009;33(Suppl 3): S158–73.

27. Szkaradkiewicz A, Marciniak R, Chudzicka-Strugala I, et al. Proinflammatory cytokines and IL-10 in inflammatory bowel disease and colorectal cancer patients. Arch Immunol Ther Exp 2009;57(4):291–4.

28. Harries AD, Beeching NJ, Rogerson SJ, et al. The platelet count as a simple measure to distinguish inflammatory bowel disease from infective diarrhoea. J Infect 1991;22(3):247–50.

29. Kapsoritakis AN, Koukourakis MI, Sfiridaki A, et al. Mean platelet volume: a useful marker of inflammatory bowel disease activity. Am J Gastroenterol 2001;96(3):776–81.

30. Song CS, Park DI, Yoon MY, et al. Association between red cell distribution width and disease activity in patients with inflammatory bowel disease. Dig Dis Sci 2012;57(4):1033–8.

31. Cracowski JL, Bonaz B, Bessard G, et al. Increased urinary F2-isoprostanes in patients with Crohn's disease. Am J Gastroenterol 2002;97(1):99–103.

32. Stanke-Labesque F, Pofelski J, Moreau-Gaudry A, et al. Urinary leukotriene E4 excretion: a biomarker of inflammatory bowel disease activity. Inflamm Bowel Dis 2008;14(6):769–74.

33. Arai Y, Arihiro S, Matsuura T, et al. Prostaglandin E-major urinary metabolite as a reliable surrogate marker for mucosal inflammation in ulcerative colitis. Inflamm Bowel Dis 2014;20(7):1208–16.

34. Judmaier G, Meyersbach P, Weiss G, et al. The role of neopterin in assessing disease activity in Crohn's disease: classification and regression trees. Am J Gastroenterol 1993;88(5):706–11.

35. Husain N, Tokoro K, Popov JM, et al. Neopterin concentration as an index of disease activity in Crohn's disease and ulcerative colitis. J Clin Gastroenterol 2013; 47(3):246–51.

36. Lehmann FS, Burri E, Beglinger C. The role and utility of faecal markers in inflammatory bowel disease. Therap Adv Gastroenterol 2015;8(1):23–36.

37. Saverymuttu SH, Peters AM, Lavender JP, et al. Quantitative fecal indium 111-labeled leukocyte excretion in the assessment of disease in Crohn's disease. Gastroenterology 1983;85(6):1333–9.

38. Becker K, Berger M, Niederau C, et al. Individual fecal alpha 1-antitrypsin excretion reflects clinical activity in Crohn's disease but not in ulcerative colitis. Hepatogastroenterology 1999;46(28):2309–14.

39. Becker K, Niederau C, Frieling T. Fecal excretion of alpha 2-macroglobulin: a novel marker for disease activity in patients with inflammatory bowel disease. Z Gastroenterol 1999;37(7):597–605.

40. Fengming Y, Jianbing W. Biomarkers of inflammatory bowel disease. Dis Markers 2014;2014:710915.

41. Lamb CA, Mansfield JC. Measurement of faecal calprotectin and lactoferrin in inflammatory bowel disease. Frontline Gastroenterol 2011;2(1):13–8.

42. Konikoff MR, Denson LA. Role of fecal calprotectin as a biomarker of intestinal inflammation in inflammatory bowel disease. Inflamm Bowel Dis 2006;12(6):524–34.

43. Alibrahim B, Aljasser MI, Salh B. Fecal calprotectin use in inflammatory bowel disease and beyond: A mini-review. Can J Gastroenterol Hepatol 2015;29(3): 157–63.

44. Soubieres AA, Poullis A. Emerging role of novel biomarkers in the diagnosis of inflammatory bowel disease. World J Gastrointest Pharmacol Ther 2016;7(1):41–50.

45. Boon GJ, Day AS, Mulder CJ, et al. Are faecal markers good indicators of mucosal healing in inflammatory bowel disease? World J Gastroenterol 2015; 21(40):11469–80.

46. Wagner M, Peterson CG, Ridefelt P, et al. Fecal markers of inflammation used as surrogate markers for treatment outcome in relapsing inflammatory bowel disease. World J Gastroenterol 2008;14(36):5584–9 [discussion: 8].

47. Silberer H, Kuppers B, Mickisch O, et al. Fecal leukocyte proteins in inflammatory bowel disease and irritable bowel syndrome. Clin Lab 2005;51(3–4): 117–26.

48. Peterson CG, Sangfelt P, Wagner M, et al. Fecal levels of leukocyte markers reflect disease activity in patients with ulcerative colitis. Scand J Clin Lab Invest 2007;67(8):810–20.
49. Avdagic N, Zaciragic A, Babic N, et al. Nitric oxide as a potential biomarker in inflammatory bowel disease. Bosn J Basic Med Sci 2013;13(1):5–9.
50. Malerba M, Ragnoli B, Buffoli L, et al. Exhaled nitric oxide as a marker of lung involvement in Crohn's disease. Int J Immunopathol Pharmacol 2011;24(4): 1119–24.
51. Lundberg JO, Hellstrom PM, Fagerhol MK, et al. Technology insight: calprotectin, lactoferrin and nitric oxide as novel markers of inflammatory bowel disease. Nat Clin Pract Gastroenterol Hepatol 2005;2(2):96–102.
52. Reinders CI, Herulf M, Ljung T, et al. Rectal mucosal nitric oxide in differentiation of inflammatory bowel disease and irritable bowel syndrome. Clin Gastroenterol Hepatol 2005;3(8):777–83.
53. Reinders CA, Jonkers D, Janson EA, et al. Rectal nitric oxide and fecal calprotectin in inflammatory bowel disease. Scand J Gastroenterol 2007;42(10): 1151–7.
54. Ljung T, Lundberg S, Varsanyi M, et al. Rectal nitric oxide as biomarker in the treatment of inflammatory bowel disease: responders versus nonresponders. World J Gastroenterol 2006;12(21):3386–92.
55. Ho GT, Lee HM, Brydon G, et al. Fecal calprotectin predicts the clinical course of acute severe ulcerative colitis. Am J Gastroenterol 2009;104(3):673–8.
56. Rubin DT, Mulani P, Chao J, et al. Effect of adalimumab on clinical laboratory parameters in patients with Crohn's disease: results from the CHARM trial. Inflamm Bowel Dis 2012;18(5):818–25.
57. Koelewijn CL, Schwartz MP, Samsom M, et al. C-reactive protein levels during a relapse of Crohn's disease are associated with the clinical course of the disease. World J Gastroenterol 2008;14(1):85–9.
58. Cornillie F, Hanauer SB, Diamond RH, et al. Postinduction serum infliximab trough level and decrease of C-reactive protein level are associated with durable sustained response to infliximab: a retrospective analysis of the ACCENT I trial. Gut 2014;63(11):1721–7.
59. Mosli MH, Zou G, Garg SK, et al. C-reactive protein, fecal calprotectin, and stool lactoferrin for detection of endoscopic activity in symptomatic inflammatory bowel disease patients: a systematic review and meta-analysis. Am J Gastroenterol 2015;110(6):802–19 [quiz: 20].
60. D'Haens G, Ferrante M, Vermeire S, et al. Fecal calprotectin is a surrogate marker for endoscopic lesions in inflammatory bowel disease. Inflamm Bowel Dis 2012;18(12):2218–24.
61. Garcia-Sanchez V, Iglesias-Flores E, Gonzalez R, et al. Does fecal calprotectin predict relapse in patients with Crohn's disease and ulcerative colitis? J Crohns Colitis 2010;4(2):144–52.
62. Lobaton T, Lopez-Garcia A, Rodriguez-Moranta F, et al. A new rapid test for fecal calprotectin predicts endoscopic remission and postoperative recurrence in Crohn's disease. J Crohns Colitis 2013;7(12):e641–51.
63. Boschetti G, Laidet M, Moussata D, et al. Levels of fecal calprotectin are associated with the severity of postoperative endoscopic recurrence in asymptomatic patients with Crohn's disease. Am J Gastroenterol 2015;110(6):865–72.
64. Wright EK, Kamm MA, De Cruz P, et al. Measurement of fecal calprotectin improves monitoring and detection of recurrence of Crohn's disease after surgery. Gastroenterology 2015;148(5):938–47.e1.

65. Yamamoto T, Shimoyama T, Bamba T, et al. Consecutive monitoring of fecal cal-protectin and lactoferrin for the early diagnosis and prediction of pouchitis after restorative proctocolectomy for ulcerative colitis. Am J Gastroenterol 2015; 110(6):881–7.

66. van Rheenen PF, Van de Vijver E, Fidler V. Faecal calprotectin for screening of patients with suspected inflammatory bowel disease: diagnostic meta-analysis. BMJ 2010;341:c3369.

67. Menees SB, Powell C, Kurlander J, et al. A meta-analysis of the utility of C-reactive protein, erythrocyte sedimentation rate, fecal calprotectin, and fecal lactoferrin to exclude inflammatory bowel disease in adults with IBS. Am J Gastroenterol 2015; 110(3):444–54.

68. Schoepfer AM, Beglinger C, Straumann A, et al. Fecal calprotectin correlates more closely with the Simple Endoscopic Score for Crohn's disease (SES-CD) than CRP, blood leukocytes, and the CDAI. Am J Gastroenterol 2010;105(1): 162–9.

69. Benitez JM, Garcia-Sanchez V. Faecal calprotectin: management in inflamma-tory bowel disease. World J Gastrointest Pathophysiol 2015;6(4):203–9.

70. Schoepfer AM, Beglinger C, Straumann A, et al. Fecal calprotectin more accu-rately reflects endoscopic activity of ulcerative colitis than the Lichtiger Index, C-reactive protein, platelets, hemoglobin, and blood leukocytes. Inflamm Bowel Dis 2013;19(2):332–41.

71. Guardiola J, Lobaton T, Rodriguez-Alonso L, et al. Fecal level of calprotectin identifies histologic inflammation in patients with ulcerative colitis in clinical and endoscopic remission. Clin Gastroenterol Hepatol 2014;12(11):1865–70.

72. Cerrillo E, Beltran B, Pous S, et al. Fecal calprotectin in ileal Crohn's disease: relationship with magnetic resonance enterography and a pathology score. In-flamm Bowel Dis 2015;21(7):1572–9.

73. Koulaouzidis A, Sipponen T, Nemeth A, et al. Association between fecal calpro-tectin levels and small-bowel inflammation score in capsule endoscopy: a multi-center retrospective study. Dig Dis Sci 2016;61(7):2033–40.

74. Henriksen M, Jahnsen J, Lygren I, et al. C-reactive protein: a predictive factor and marker of inflammation in inflammatory bowel disease. Results from a pro-spective population-based study. Gut 2008;57(11):1518–23.

75. Solem CA, Loftus EV Jr, Tremaine WJ, et al. Correlation of C-reactive protein with clinical, endoscopic, histologic, and radiographic activity in inflammatory bowel disease. Inflamm Bowel Dis 2005;11(8):707–12.

76. af Bjorkesten CG, Nieminen U, Turunen U, et al. Surrogate markers and clinical indices, alone or combined, as indicators for endoscopic remission in anti-TNF-treated luminal Crohn's disease. Scand J Gastroenterol 2012;47(5):528–37.

77. Costa F, Mumolo MG, Ceccarelli L, et al. Calprotectin is a stronger predictive marker of relapse in ulcerative colitis than in Crohn's disease. Gut 2005;54(3): 364–8.

78. D'Inca R, Dal Pont E, Di Leo V, et al. Can calprotectin predict relapse risk in in-flammatory bowel disease? Am J Gastroenterol 2008;103(8):2007–14.

79. Ferreiro-Iglesias R, Barreiro-de Acosta M, Otero Santiago M, et al. Fecal calpro-tectin as predictor of relapse in patients with inflammatory bowel disease under maintenance infliximab therapy. J Clin Gastroenterol 2016;50(2):147–51.

80. Ferreiro-Iglesias R, Barreiro-de Acosta M, Lorenzo-Gonzalez A, et al. Useful-ness of a rapid faecal calprotectin test to predict relapse in Crohn's disease pa-tients on maintenance treatment with adalimumab. Scand J Gastroenterol 2016; 51(4):442–7.

81. Bitton A, Dobkin PL, Edwardes MD, et al. Predicting relapse in Crohn's disease: a biopsychosocial model. Gut 2008;57(10):1386–92.

82. Osterman MT, Aberra FN, Cross R, et al. Mesalamine dose escalation reduces fecal calprotectin in patients with quiescent ulcerative colitis. Clin Gastroenterol Hepatol 2014;12(11):1887–93.e3.

83. Kolho KL, Raivio T, Lindahl H, et al. Fecal calprotectin remains high during glucocorticoid therapy in children with inflammatory bowel disease. Scand J Gastroenterol 2006;41(6):720–5.

84. De Vos M, Dewit O, D'Haens G, et al. Fast and sharp decrease in calprotectin predicts remission by infliximab in anti-TNF naive patients with ulcerative colitis. J Crohns Colitis 2012;6(5):557–62.

85. Peyrin-Biroulet L, Reinisch W, Colombel JF, et al. Clinical disease activity, C-reactive protein normalisation and mucosal healing in Crohn's disease in the SONIC trial. Gut 2014;63(1):88–95.

86. Gelbmann CM. Prediction of treatment refractoriness in ulcerative colitis and Crohn's disease–do we have reliable markers? Inflamm Bowel Dis 2000;6(2): 123–31.

87. Magro F, Rodrigues-Pinto E, Santos-Antunes J, et al. High C-reactive protein in Crohn's disease patients predicts nonresponse to infliximab treatment. J Crohns Colitis 2014;8(2):129–36.

88. Karmiris K, Paintaud G, Noman M, et al. Influence of trough serum levels and immunogenicity on long-term outcome of adalimumab therapy in Crohn's disease. Gastroenterology 2009;137(5):1628–40.

89. Jurgens M, Mahachie John JM, Cleynen I, et al. Levels of C-reactive protein are associated with response to infliximab therapy in patients with Crohn's disease. Clin Gastroenterol Hepatol 2011;9(5):421–7.e1.

90. Kiss LS, Szamosi T, Molnar T, et al. Early clinical remission and normalisation of CRP are the strongest predictors of efficacy, mucosal healing and dose escalation during the first year of adalimumab therapy in Crohn's disease. Aliment Pharmacol Ther 2011;34(8):911–22.

91. Hibi T, Sakuraba A, Watanabe M, et al. C-reactive protein is an indicator of serum infliximab level in predicting loss of response in patients with Crohn's disease. J Gastroenterol 2014;49(2):254–62.

92. Lamb CA, Mohiuddin MK, Gicquel J, et al. Faecal calprotectin or lactoferrin can identify postoperative recurrence in Crohn's disease. Br J Surg 2009;96(6): 663–74.

93. Orlando A, Modesto I, Castiglione F, et al. The role of calprotectin in predicting endoscopic post-surgical recurrence in asymptomatic Crohn's disease: a comparison with ultrasound. Eur Rev Med Pharmacol Sci 2006;10(1):17–22.

94. De Cruz P, Kamm MA, Hamilton AL, et al. Crohn's disease management after intestinal resection: a randomised trial. Lancet 2015;385(9976):1406–17.

95. Regueiro M, Kip KE, Schraut W, et al. Crohn's disease activity index does not correlate with endoscopic recurrence one year after ileocolonic resection. Inflamm Bowel Dis 2011;17(1):118–26.

96. Sorrentino D, Paviotti A, Terrosu G, et al. Low-dose maintenance therapy with infliximab prevents postsurgical recurrence of Crohn's disease. Clin Gastroenterol Hepatol 2010;8(7):591–9.e1 [quiz: e78–9].

97. Pakarinen MP, Koivusalo A, Natunen J, et al. Fecal calprotectin mirrors inflammation of the distal ileum and bowel function after restorative proctocolectomy for pediatric-onset ulcerative colitis. Inflamm Bowel Dis 2010;16(3):482–6.

98. Johnson MW, Maestranzi S, Duffy AM, et al. Faecal calprotectin: a noninvasive diagnostic tool and marker of severity in pouchitis. Eur J Gastroenterol Hepatol 2008;20(3):174–9.

99. McGovern DP, Kugathasan S, Cho JH. Genetics of inflammatory bowel diseases. Gastroenterology 2015;149(5):1163–76.e2.

100. Iborra M, Bernuzzi F, Correale C, et al. Identification of serum and tissue microRNA expression profiles in different stages of inflammatory bowel disease. Clin Exp Immunol 2013;173(2):250–8.

101. Chapman CG, Pekow J. The emerging role of miRNAs in inflammatory bowel disease: a review. Therap Adv Gastroenterol 2015;8(1):4–22.

102. Kalla R, Ventham NT, Kennedy NA. MicroRNAs: new players in inflammatory bowel disease. Gut 2015;64(6):1008.

103. Bennike T, Birkelund S, Stensballe A, et al. Biomarkers in inflammatory bowel diseases: current status and proteomics identification strategies. World J Gastroenterol 2014;20(12):3231–44.

104. Markar SR, Wiggins T, Kumar S, et al. Exhaled breath analysis for the diagnosis and assessment of endoluminal gastrointestinal diseases. J Clin Gastroenterol 2015;49(1):1–8.

105. Kurada S, Alkhouri N, Fiocchi C, et al. Review article: breath analysis in inflammatory bowel diseases. Aliment Pharmacol Ther 2015;41(4):329–41.

Endomicroscopy and Molecular Tools to Evaluate Inflammatory Bowel Disease

Anna M. Buchner, MD, PhD[a], Michael B. Wallace, MD, MPH[b],*

KEYWORDS

- Confocal endomicroscopy • Colonoscopy • Ulcerative colitis • Crohn's disease
- Inflammatory assessment • Dysplasia • Molecular imaging

KEY POINTS

- Confocal laser endomicroscopy (CLE) is a rapidly emerging tool in endoscopic imaging allowing in vivo microscopy of examined gastrointestinal mucosa. CLE also has the potential to enhance the endoscopic evaluation of inflammatory bowel disease (IBD). This may be achieved by further characterization of otherwise normal-appearing mucosa, assessment of the barrier function of the epithelium, and characterization of any mucosal lesions including dysplastic lesions.
- Imaging of intestinal inflammation in IBD by CLE may be of special importance not just for the diagnosis of IBD, assessment of severity of inflammation but also for predicting severity and the guidance of therapy. This would represent a true advantage of CLE over the conventional white-light endoscopy in evaluation of IBD and assessment of a true mucosal healing.
- Advances in IBD may be used not only to better understand the pathophysiology of IBD but also to guide optimized therapy and thus allow a completely new, personalized approach to the IBD management.
- Further studies are needed to fully evaluate and validate the promising results of CLE studies in IBD.

Disclosures: None (A.M. Buchner); Receives research funding from Olympus, Ninepoint medical, Cosmo Pharmaceuticals, Boston Scientific. Honoraria from Olympus, Equity Interest in iLumen (M.B. Wallace).
[a] Division of Gastroenterology, University of Pennsylvania, 3400 Civic Center PCAM 7 South, Philadelphia, PA 19104, USA; [b] Division of Gastroenterology and Hepatology, Mayo Clinic, 4500 San Pablo Road, Jacksonville, FL 32224, USA
* Corresponding author.
E-mail address: Wallace.michael@mayo.edu

Gastrointest Endoscopy Clin N Am 26 (2016) 657–668
http://dx.doi.org/10.1016/j.giec.2016.06.002

giendo.theclinics.com

INTRODUCTION

Endoscopy is an essential tool in effective evaluation of patients with inflammatory bowel disease (IBD). The endoscopic evaluation of IBD includes not only diagnosing the disease, assessing the disease's extent and activity, but also treating its complications, monitoring the responses to treatment with evaluating mucosal healing, and serving as a predictor of disease course. The small-field endoscopic imaging technology, such as confocal laser endomicroscopy (CLE) has allowed real-time imaging of gastrointestinal mucosal during ongoing endoscopic evaluation in various gastrointestinal pathologies.[1-4] It also has the potential to enhance endoscopic evaluation in IBD. CLE is based on tissue illumination with a low-power laser allowing micron-level spatial resolution with ×1000 magnification. To obtain images, exogenous fluorescence contrast is applied with agents such as fluorescein (10% 5 mL solution, intravenous application), or acriflavine hydrochloride or cresyl violet (topical applications). Intravenous fluorescein (1.0–5.0 mL of 10% solution) distributes throughout the capillary network and connective matrix and has been universally applied in all confocal studies and is found to be generally safe in use.[5] Until recently, CLE has been performed using 1 of 2 Food and Drug Administration (FDA)-approved devices: endoscope-based confocal laser endomicroscopy (Pentax, Fort Wayne, NJ; herein termed eCLE) and a stand-alone probe CLE (herein termed pCLE) capable of passage through the accessory channel of most endoscopes (Cellvizio, Mauna Kea Technologies, Paris, France).[6] Currently the eCLE system is no longer clinically available, although most clinical applications have been studied based on that system.

The probe-based CLE system (pCLE), introduced in 2005, consists of a stand-alone confocal probe, capable of passage through an accessory channel of most endoscopes. The probe is made of 30,000 optical fibers bundled together with a distal lens and a proximal precision connector. The proximal connector attaches the probe to the laser scanning unit that is connected to a standard computer for image data processing and display (**Fig. 1**). **Table 1** lists the features of the 2 CLE systems: the current probe based and the prior endoscope based.

The value of CLE in evaluation of conditions such as Barrett esophagus, colorectal polyps, and celiac disease has been demonstrated and validated in various studies.[3,7–9] CLE also has the potential to enhance the endoscopic evaluation of IBD. This may be achieved by further characterization of the barrier function of the epithelium, assessment of inflammatory activity, characterization of any mucosal lesions, and ultimately predicting severity, disease extent, and response to the treatment.[10,11] Imaging of intestinal inflammation in IBD by CLE may be of special importance not just for the diagnosis of IBD but also for the guidance of therapy. Furthermore, advances in molecular in vivo imaging in IBD may be used to better understand the pathophysiology of IBD and to guide an optimized therapy.[12] This review discusses the most recent advances and potential applications of confocal endomicroscopy and molecular tools in the evaluation of IBD.

CONFOCAL LASER ENDOMICROSCOPY FOR ASSESSMENT OF INFLAMMATION, BARRIER FUNCTION OF EPITHELIUM, AND DISEASE RELAPSE

As the field of IBD therapy has moved to a "treat-to-target" approach, with the goal of suppressing microscopic inflammation, CLE may play an important role in assessing disease activity with detection of all inflammatory features, assessing the degree of inflammation as well as evaluating the barrier function of the epithelium.[10] CLE may also facilitate the distinction between ulcerative colitis (UC) and Crohn's disease (CD).[13]

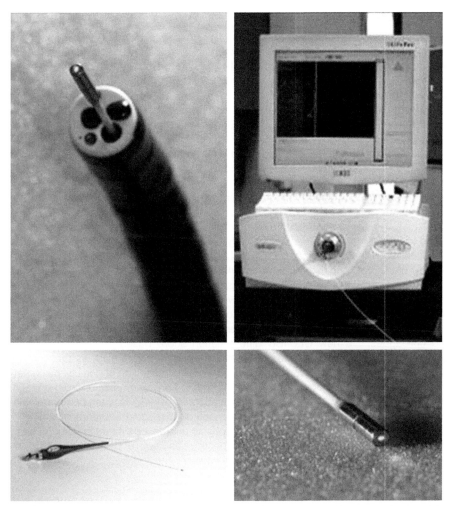

Fig. 1. Confocal microscopy probe-based system. Cellvizio, MKT, Paris, France. (*From* ASGE Technology Committee, Chauhan S, Abu Dayyeh BK, et al. Technology status evaluation report: confocal laser endomicroscopy. Gastrointest Endosc 2014;80:928-938; with permission.)

Table 1 Comparison of confocal laser endomicroscopy (CLE) systems		
System	Current System: Probe-Based CLE (pCLE) (Cellvizio, Mauna Kea Technologies, Paris, France)	Prior System: Endoscope-Based CLE (eCLE) (Pentax, Japan)
Magnification	1000 times	1000 times
Lateral Resolution	>1 μm	<1 μm
Field of view	240–600 μm	475 × 475 μm
Imaging plane depth	40–130 μm (fixed)	0–250 μm (variable)

Assessment of Inflammation and Mucosal Healing

As compared with healthy mucosa, inflamed mucosa in IBD on CLE examination has been noted for irregular and tortuous crypt with irregular and wider lumens.[11,14] In addition, an increased density of epithelial gaps and fluorescein leakage to the interstitial space also has been detected by CLE in IBD.[15–17] This is in contrast to noninflamed mucosa in which epithelium functions as an intact barrier not allowing fluorescein leakage and crypts are round and regular with small round lumina. CLE may identify IBD-associated histologic changes in macroscopically noninflamed mucosa. The new classification of pCLE in IBD to predict histologic inflammation in noninflamed-appearing mucosa based on different vessel and crypt categories was developed and validated by Neumann and colleagues[18] with an overall acceptable accuracy of 87%.

Endoscopic assessment of mucosal healing in IBD has been recognized as an important measure of disease activity, therapeutic goal, and prognostic factor. Mace and colleagues,[19] in their recent control study of 12 patients with UC in remission (UC-IR), aimed to determine whether endoscopically normal mucosa can be also confirmed by CLE to have fully resolved inflammation. Although in control patients CLE demonstrated normal colon crypts and microvessels, colonic mucosa of patients with UC-IR was noted to have impaired crypt regeneration, persistent inflammation, and increased vascular permeability. Thus, CLE imaging may allow a more adequate assessment of mucosal healing in IBD. Further studies are needed to validate these initial observations. Furthermore, CLE may help to differentiate between UC and CD. In the recent study by Tontini and colleagues,[20] a new CLE-IBD differentiation score based on endomicroscopy assessment (IDEA) has been introduced evaluating parameters such as presence or absence of architecture distortion, irregular surface, decreased crypt density, discontinuous crypt architectural abnormality, focal cryptitis, and discontinuous inflammation. The IDEA score was shown to have excellent accuracy of 93.7% when compared with the historical clinical diagnosis and the histopathological gold standard diagnosis.[20] CLE was able to visualize several disease-specific microscopic features used in standard histopathology, although due to limited penetration depth of CLE, subtle submucosal details and granulomas could not be evaluated.[20]

Assessment of Degree of Inflammation and Disease Activity

The correlation between CLE features of the crypts and the inflammation assessed by regular histopathology has been specifically examined in recent studies in patients with UC and patients with CD.[21–23] The Chang–Quing scale has been introduced assessing the degree of inflammation based on the crypt architecture: the regularity of crypt arrangement, crypt density, dilation of crypt lumens, and crypt destruction and subsequently validated by comparison with endoscopic assessment and clinical outcomes in UC.[21,24] Li and colleagues[21] demonstrated good correlation between CLE assessment of crypt architecture and fluorescein leakage with histologic results in patients with UC. Interestingly, more than half of the patients with normal mucosa seen on conventional white-light endoscopy showed acute inflammation on histology, whereas no patients with normal mucosa or with chronic inflammation seen on CLE showed acute inflammation on histology.[21] Assessment of microvascular alteration by CLE also showed good correlation with histologic finings.[21] The presence of fluorescein leakage correlated with histologic assessment of inflammation.[21,22] The additional studies in UC compared the CLE-documented inflammation with histopathology assessment.[21,22] Based on those studies, the CLE assessment of crypts' architecture strongly correlated with the degree of inflammation assessed by histology, while higher level of fluorescein leakage was noted in active disease as compared with quiescent disease. Buda and colleagues[22] divided patients with UC into 3 groups depending on a composite outcome score combining the amount of fluorescein leakage and crypt diameters and determined that this composite outcome score was able to predict a disease flare during a 12-month follow-up period ($P < .01$). Specifically depending on each group's score, relapse rate ranged from 6 of 7, 1 of 6, and 0 of 6 during the following year.

Based on those studies, the crypt architecture, microvascular alteration, and fluorescein leakage can represent promising markers in CLE evaluation of IBD, although further studies validating these initial observations are required.

Neumann and colleagues[23] evaluated CLE features of inflamed mucosa in patients with CD. The Crohn's Disease Endomicroscopic Activity Score (CDEAS) to evaluate CD colitis activity in vivo (active vs nonactive) was developed in a prospective study of 54 patients with CD using eCLE and pCLE.[23] The CDEAS included parameters such as crypt number (increased, decreased), colonic crypt distortion microerosions, augmented vascularization, number of goblet cells (increased or decreased), and increased cellular infiltration within lamina propria. By assigning 1 point for each given parameter, the total score ranged from 0 to 8.[23] Quiescent CD colitis was noted to have a significant increase in crypt and goblet cell numbers with median CDEAS score of 2, whereas patients with active colitis had a score of 5. There was also significant association of the CDEAS score with inflammatory markers, such as C-reactive protein, but further associations with histology, endoscopic assessment, and clinical outcomes are to be established.

In addition, the Watson grading system has been introduced and based on parameters such as fluorescein leakage to the lumen of the small intestine and the presence of microerosions.[15,25] The system has been also compared with the clinical outcomes but not endoscopic or histologic assessment of IBD.[15,25] **Table 2** compares all available the CLE-based systems for the inflammation assessment in IBD.

Assessment of Epithelial Barrier Function and Disease Relapse

CLE has been used to assess gastrointestinal (GI) barrier function in the study by Kiesslich and colleagues.[25] Defects in intestinal barrier function of epithelial cells and the tight junction have been associated with intestinal IBD and increased intestinal permeability has been determined as a prognostic indicator of relapse.[26] Using this technique, Kiesslich and colleagues[25] demonstrated that they could detect single-cell shedding and barrier loss in the terminal ileum of patients with IBD and therefore predict relapse. Specifically CLE was used in detecting shedding epithelial cells and local barrier defects with fluorescein effluxing through the epithelium. Mouse experiments confirmed inward flow through some leakage-associated shedding events, which was increased when luminal osmolarity was decreased.[25] Interestingly, in patients with IBD in clinical remission, this increased cell shedding with fluorescein leakage was associated with subsequent relapse within 12 months after endomicroscopic examination ($P < .001$) The sensitivity, specificity, and accuracy of this grading system to predict a flare of 62.5% (95% confidence interval [CI] 40.8%–80.4%), 91.2% (95% CI 75.2%–97.7%), and 79% (95% CI 57.7%–95.5%), respectively. This represents truly great potential of the utilization of the CLE system in predicting the disease course and a subsequent relapse. Similarly, Lim and colleagues[15] also noted that CLE can detect epithelial damage and barrier loss in the duodenum of patients with UC and CD that is not apparent on conventional endoscopic evaluation. Based on the study, patients with CD and patients with UC had significantly more epithelial

Table 2
Confocal laser endomicroscopy–based rating systems of the degree of inflammation and prediction of the relapse

CLE Grading Systems	Degree of Assessed Changes with Specific Features	Relapse Prediction
Chang-Qing system[21] based on pCLE in UC, validated with respect to histology, endoscopic assessment, and clinical outcomes	A: No inflammation: regular size and arrangement of the crypts B: Chronic inflammation: enlarges space between crypts and irregular crypt architecture C: Acute inflammation: crypt openings enlarged, more irregular architecture of the crypts with enlargement of the space between crypts, more than grade B D: Acute inflammation: severe crypt destruction and/or crypt abscesses	Prediction of relapse by histologic criteria of acute inflammation with regard to sensitivity, specificity, accuracy was 71%, 90%, and 79% When using CLE criteria of acute inflammation, sensitivity, specificity, and accuracy of 64%, 89%, and 74%
Watson grading system in CD and UC based on eCLE and pCLE[15,25]	I: Normal: single-cell shedding with no barrier dysfunction II: Functional defect with cell shedding confined to single cells per shedding site and visible fluorescein signal III: Structural defects: miroerosions defined when the lamina propria is exposed to the lumen with numerous cells shed per site: Intense fluorescein signal, leakage of fluorescein	Watson score of 2 or 3 had a sensitivity of 63% and specificity of 91% for the prediction of relapse within 12 months[25]
CD Endomicroscopic Activity Score (CDEAS) in CD based on eCLE and pCLE	I: Quiescent CD based on increased/decrease of crypt number, crypt lumen, tortuosity, microerosions, vascularity, goblet cell, cellular infiltrate II: Active CD based on increased/decrease of crypt number, crypt lumen, tortuosity, microerosions, vascularity, goblet cell, cellular infiltrate	Not validated with histology, endoscopic assessment, clinical symptoms

Abbreviations: CD, Crohn's disease; CLE, confocal laser endomicroscopy; eCLE, endoscope-based CLE; pCLE, probe-based CLE; UC, ulcerative colitis.

gaps, epithelial cell shedding, and leakage of fluorescein into the duodenal lumen than controls. The degree of cell shedding and epithelial gap formation was similar in patients with CD and patients with UC. In all cases, macroscopic endoscopic appearances of the duodenum were normal, and conventional histologic analysis showed a mild nonspecific duodenitis in 7 of 15 patients with CD. Patients with UC had a histologically normal duodenum. Gap formation, cell shedding, and fluorescein leakage was similar in CD with active compared with inactive disease.

CLE has been also applied to visualize intramucosal enteric bacteria in vivo in patients with IBD. Intramucosal bacteria were confirmed to be found more frequently and with a wider distribution in patients with IBD than in patients with a normal intestine.[27] These studies suggest that CLE may offer an important method to improve our understanding of bacterial translocation, epithelial shedding, and loss of GI barrier leading to improved diagnostic and treatment capabilities in these challenging conditions.

CONFOCAL LASER ENDOMICROSCOPY FOR DYSPLASIA SURVEILLANCE IN INFLAMMATORY BOWEL DISEASE
Confocal Laser Endomicroscopy for Colitis-Associated Dysplasia and Colorectal Cancer in Inflammatory Bowel Disease

The incidence of UC and CD has been rising.[28] Patients with these conditions are at higher risk for the development of colitis-associated colorectal cancer. In the chronic IBD setting, CLE systems can be used in combination with one of the red-flag techniques, such as traditional dye-based chromoendoscopy or virtual chromoendoscopy (eg, Narrow band imaging [NBI], I-Scan, Fujifilm intelligent chromo-endoscopy [FICE]) for the initial detection and characterization of subtle mucosal abnormalities and circumscribed lesions. Once the targeted lesion or mucosal abnormality is detected, it can then be interrogated further by the confocal system for in vivo histology (**Fig. 2**). To date, various studies have examined the potential role of CLE in IBD surveillance, suggesting that this technique can have an important role in targeting biopsies to improve the early detection of neoplasia and dysplasia characterization.[29–31] Kiesslich and colleagues[29] showed that by using chromoendoscopy with endomicroscopy (eCLE), the detection of neoplasia increased 4.75-fold, with 50% fewer biopsies required. The presence of neoplastic changes in the settings of IBD could be predicted by endomicroscopy with high accuracy (sensitivity 94.7%; specificity 98.3%; accuracy 97.8%).[29]

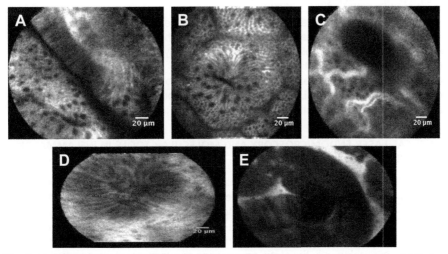

Fig. 2. Endoscopic confocal images of colon in IBD. (*A*) Normal colon mucosa. (*B*) Colon crypt. (*C*) Colonic vasculature. (*D*) Colonic inflammation with crypt fusion/distortion and increased vasculature, (*E*) Colonic dysplasia with increased epithelial density, irregular crypts, and increased vasculature.

The study by Gunther and colleagues[32] reviewed different endoscopic strategies for neoplasia detection in the setting of IBD and concluded that eCLE-targeted biopsies led to much higher detection of neoplasia compared with random biopsies alone.

In contrast, a Dutch study by Van den Broek and colleagues[33] evaluated the feasibility and found the diagnostic accuracy of pCLE to be much lower, with an estimated accuracy, sensitivity, and specificity of 81%, 65%, and 82%, respectively. Prolongation of the procedure by 30 minutes was noted, as well as the presence of good and excellent image quality in only 69% of patients with the use of pCLE.

The recent systematic review and meta-analysis evaluating the overall efficacy of all CLE systems for discriminating colorectal neoplasia, including patients with IBD, concluded that CLE is comparable to colonoscopy histopathology in diagnosing colorectal neoplasia (overall CLE sensitivity and specificity was 0.93 and 0.97 specificity, for IBD subgroup sensitivity was 0.83 and specificity 0.90).[34] For real-time CLE, endoscopy-based systems had better sensitivity (0.97 vs 0.82, $P < .001$) and specificity (0.99 vs 0.82, $P < .001$) than probe-based systems.[34]

The most recent study by Wanders and colleagues[35] evaluated the diagnostic accuracy of chromoendoscopy combined with endoscope-based confocal microscopy for dysplasia diagnosis in CD colitis and confirmed overall good accuracy but low sensitivities in distinguishing dysplastic versus nondysplastic lesions. This is in contrast to the prior initial studies reporting much higher estimates of accuracy, sensitivity, and specificity.[29,34] Those differences raise questions about the future applications of this technology. The evaluation of dysplastic lesions by CLE can be challenging especially in the background of regeneration and inflammatory changes, and inflammatory lesions can be easily misread as dysplastic or dysplastic lesions reported as nondysplastic. Reported failure of eCLE equipment resulted in terminating the study earlier and since then eCLE has been withdrawn completely from commercial use. Thus, the role of alternative and currently the only available CLE system, pCLE, for dysplasia surveillance is still to be determined.

Confocal Laser Endomicroscopy for Dysplasia in Patients with Inflammatory Bowel Disease/Primary Sclerosing Cholangitis

CLE also has been suggested as a diagnostic tool for evaluation of biliary dysplasia in patients with primary sclerosing cholangitis (PSC).[36] The recent study by Heif and colleagues[36] evaluating the role of pCLE in excluding dysplasia of dominant strictures confirmed 100% sensitivity, 60% specificity, and negative predictive value of 100%.[36] Furthermore, patients with PSC/IBD are also known to have a high risk for colorectal cancer; thus, pCLE may be an important tool in enhancing dysplasia evaluation in these high-risk patients.

CONFOCAL LASER ENDOMICROSCOPY AND MOLECULAR TOOLS IN INFLAMMATORY BOWEL DISEASE

CLE also has been used for molecular imaging, which has the potential to enhance detection of disease-specific morphologic or functional tissue alterations and help to provide molecular-targeted therapies. Molecular imaging uses fluorescently labeled probes (antibodies or peptides) to highlight abnormal lesions based on their molecular signatures. Molecular imaging relies on visualization of biological properties of a lesion rather than assessing only the static appearance of a lesion and aims to evaluate the potential response to targeted therapy. Such molecular imaging has been successfully used in animal models of gut inflammation and cancer, in vivo and ex vivo. Various point-targeted endomicroscopic devices have been used to characterize the lesion and visualize the in vivo interaction of targeted drugs within the lesion. This potential has been demonstrated in a study by Hsiung and colleagues[37] aiming to develop a probe for detecting colon cancer, using a phage peptide library against fresh human colonic adenomas to screen for high-affinity ligands with preferential binding to premalignant tissue and using the CLE system during colonoscopy.[37] A specific heptapeptide sequence conjugated with fluorescein was identified and tested subsequently through topical application in patients undergoing colonoscopy.[37] It was demonstrated that the fluorescein-conjugated peptide bound more strongly to dysplastic colonocytes than to adjacent normal cells, with 81% sensitivity and 82% specificity. This methodology represents a promising diagnostic imaging approach for the early detection of colorectal cancer and potentially of other epithelial malignancies.[37]

Goetz and colleagues[38] demonstrated the applicability of endomicroscopy for in vivo molecular imaging of epidermal growth factor receptors (EGFR) of human xenograft tumors in mice. CLE could identify EGFR expression accurately after injection of fluorescently labeled antibodies against EGFR. The same group has further demonstrated the potential for CLE as a prediction tool for molecular therapy in colorectal cancer, showing that the binding of the anti-EGFR monoclonal antibody, cetuximab, to xenographs of colon cancer cells as imaged by CLE predicted the response to therapeutic doses of cetuximab in a mouse model of colorectal cancer.[39]

The recent human in vivo study by Schmidt and colleagues[40] evaluated the role of nanoscaled and microscaled particles for drug targeting to inflamed intestinal mucosa in patients with IBD. In their experiment, after rectal application of florescent-labeled placebo nanoparticles and microparticles to 33 patients with IBD and controls, CLE was used to visualize the particles in inflamed areas. There was a significant accumulation of microparticles in ulcerated lesions, whereas nanoparticles were only minimally visible in the mucosal surface of all patients. This led to the conclusion that nanoparticles may not be required for local drug delivery to intestinal lesions in humans.

Atreya and colleagues[41] analyzed the response to biological treatment with anti–tumor necrosis factor (TNF) therapy using in vivo molecular imaging. Topical administration of fluorescent anti-TNF (adalimumab) in 25 patients with CD led to the detection of intestinal membrane-bound TNF$^-$ mTNF$^+$ immune cells during CLE examination. Based on quantitative image analysis, patients could be clearly divided into 2 groups: high mTNF versus low mTNF. Patients with high numbers of mTNF$^+$ cells had significantly higher short-term clinical response rates (92%) at week 12 on subsequent anti-TNF therapy compared with patients with low amounts of mTNF$^+$ cells (15%).[41] These findings imply that molecular imaging with fluorescent anti-TNF permits prediction of clinical responses to anti-TNF therapy. This may facilitate early patient stratification in choosing therapeutic approaches. Larger prospective studies are still required to fully validate these promising results. However, the exciting new era has begun with our endoscopic imaging being moved beyond being simply a diagnostic tool to becoming a prediction tool for molecular therapies, guiding the treatment of our patients, assessing efficacy of biological treatment, and providing personalized therapy approaches in IBD.

SUMMARY

In summary, confocal endomicroscopy represents a truly promising advance in IBDs. It may provide not only histology in vivo with an assessment of inflammatory activity, but also has potential to further visualize the ongoing pathophysiological process at the microscopic level and to apply molecular imaging to directly guide medical therapies in the future. It may further enhance surveillance of dysplasia in IBD with the use of microscopic-guided biopsies ("smart biopsies") where the yield of conventional random biopsies for dysplasia is very low.

As detailed in the most recent systemic review of all CLE studies in IBD, various clinical applications of endomicroscopy in IBD evaluation have been explored assessing the degree of inflammation, predicting the relapse and therapeutic response as well as enhancing dysplasia detection and characterization among patients with IBD undergoing endoscopic evaluation.[10]

Neumann and colleagues[42] confirmed an overall short learning curve for pCLE in patients with IBD, concluding that in general CLE may be an easy-to-learn tool for in vivo assessment of IBD. As of today, CLE remains used primarily in academic centers as an experimental tool and it has not been included in the any official guidelines on the evaluation of IBD. However, this is the only method that allows in vivo functional assessment of intestinal epithelium and barrier function in IBD and thus it represents a very promising tool for IBD evaluation. However, overall, although promising, CLE technologies have not been found to be universally accurate, with variation of results among confocal studies depending on the use of confocal systems eCLE versus pCLE.[10,29,33,35] There is definitely a need for more studies exploring and further validating the accuracy and application of the currently only available pCLE system. Moreover, the cost of pCLE technology, still high compared with a traditional histology examination, remains an important concern. More durable and less expensive confocal probes are needed for this technology to become more available in GI IBD practices.

In conclusion, CLE technology is currently a promising advance in the field of IBD. Even though many applications of this technology have proved to be feasible and clinically relevant when performed in expert hands in other GI entities such as post-endoscopic mucosal resection (EMR) scars, colorectal polyps, Barrett esophagus, CLE applications in IBD, including physiologic and molecular imaging in IBD, need to be explored and further validated.[4] Thus, as of today, CLE remains used in only selective IBD academic centers as a primarily research tool and has not yet been incorporated into standard GI guidelines of IBD management.

REFERENCES

1. Wallace MB, Fockens P. Probe-based confocal laser endomicroscopy. Gastroenterology 2009;136:1509–13.
2. Buchner AM, Shahid MW, Heckman MG, et al. Comparison of probe-based confocal laser endomicroscopy with virtual chromoendoscopy for classification of colon polyps. Gastroenterology 2010;138:834–42.
3. Dunbar K, Canto M. Confocal endomicroscopy. Curr Opin Gastroenterol 2008;24: 631–7.
4. Committee AT. Confocal laser endomicroscopy. Gastrointest Endosc 2014;80: 928–38.
5. Wallace MB, Meining A, Canto MI, et al. The safety of intravenous fluorescein for confocal laser endomicroscopy in the gastrointestinal tract. Aliment Pharmacol Ther 2010;31:548–52.
6. Kiesslich R, Goetz M, Neurath MF. Virtual histology. Best Pract Res Clin Gastroenterol 2008;22:883–97.
7. Goetz M, Kiesslich R. Confocal endomicroscopy: in vivo diagnosis of neoplastic lesions of the gastrointestinal tract. Anticancer Res 2008;28:353–60.
8. Kiesslich R, Goetz M, Vieth M, et al. Technology insight: confocal laser endoscopy for in vivo diagnosis of colorectal cancer. Nat Clin Pract Oncol 2007;4:480–90.

9. Wang KK, Carr-Locke DL, Singh SK, et al. Use of probe-based confocal laser endomicroscopy (pCLE) in gastrointestinal applications. A consensus report based on clinical evidence. United Eur Gastroenterol J 2015;3:230–54.

10. Rasmussen DN, Karstensen JG, Riis LB, et al. Confocal laser endomicroscopy in inflammatory bowel disease–a systematic review. J Crohns Colitis 2015;9: 1152–9.

11. Watanabe O, Ando T, Maeda O, et al. Confocal endomicroscopy in patients with ulcerative colitis. J Gastroenterol Hepatol 2008;23(Suppl 2):S286–90.

12. Neurath MF. Molecular endoscopy and in vivo imaging in inflammatory bowel diseases. Dig Dis 2015;33(Suppl 1):32–6.

13. Hundorfean G, Chiriac MT, Mudter J, et al. Confocal laser endomicroscopy provides potential differentiation criteria between Crohn's disease and ulcerative colitis. Inflamm Bowel Dis 2013;19:E61–4.

14. Musquer N, Coquenlorge S, Bourreille A, et al. Probe-based confocal laser endomicroscopy: a new method for quantitative analysis of pit structure in healthy and Crohn's disease patients. Dig Liver Dis 2013;45:487–92.

15. Lim LG, Neumann J, Hansen T, et al. Confocal endomicroscopy identifies loss of local barrier function in the duodenum of patients with Crohn's disease and ulcerative colitis. Inflamm Bowel Dis 2014;20:892–900.

16. Liu JJ, Madsen KL, Boulanger P, et al. Mind the gaps: confocal endomicroscopy showed increased density of small bowel epithelial gaps in inflammatory bowel disease. J Clin Gastroenterol 2011;45:240–5.

17. Liu JJ, Wong K, Thiesen AL, et al. Increased epithelial gaps in the small intestines of patients with inflammatory bowel disease: density matters. Gastrointest Endosc 2011;73:1174–80.

18. Neumann H, Coron E, Mönkemüller K, et al. Development of a new classification for confocal laser endomicroscopy in IBD. Gastrointest Endosc 2013;77(5): AB163.

19. Mace V, Ahluwalia A, Coron E, et al. Confocal laser endomicroscopy: a new gold standard for the assessment of mucosal healing in ulcerative colitis. J Gastroenterol Hepatol 2015;30(Suppl 1):85–92.

20. Tontini GE, Mudter J, Vieth M, et al. Confocal laser endomicroscopy for the differential diagnosis of ulcerative colitis and Crohn's disease: a pilot study. Endoscopy 2015;47:437–43.

21. Li CQ, Xie XJ, Yu T, et al. Classification of inflammation activity in ulcerative colitis by confocal laser endomicroscopy. Am J Gastroenterol 2010;105:1391–6.

22. Buda A, Hatem G, Neumann H, et al. Confocal laser endomicroscopy for prediction of disease relapse in ulcerative colitis: a pilot study. J Crohns Colitis 2014;8: 304–11.

23. Neumann H, Vieth M, Atreya R, et al. Assessment of Crohn's disease activity by confocal laser endomicroscopy. Inflamm Bowel Dis 2012;18:2261–9.

24. Li CQ, Liu J, Ji R, et al. Use of confocal laser endomicroscopy to predict relapse of ulcerative colitis. BMC Gastroenterol 2014;14:45.

25. Kiesslich R, Duckworth CA, Moussata D, et al. Local barrier dysfunction identified by confocal laser endomicroscopy predicts relapse in inflammatory bowel disease. Gut 2012;61:1146–53.

26. Wyatt J, Vogelsang H, Hubl W, et al. Intestinal permeability and the prediction of relapse in Crohn's disease. Lancet 1993;341:1437–9.

27. Moussata D, Goetz M, Gloeckner A, et al. Confocal laser endomicroscopy is a new imaging modality for recognition of intramucosal bacteria in inflammatory bowel disease in vivo. Gut 2011;60:26–33.

28. Lewis JD, Deren JJ, Lichtenstein GR. Cancer risk in patients with inflammatory bowel disease. Gastroenterol Clin North Am 1999;28:459–77.

29. Kiesslich R, Goetz M, Lammersdorf K, et al. Chromoscopy-guided endomicroscopy increases the diagnostic yield of intraepithelial neoplasia in ulcerative colitis. Gastroenterology 2007;132:874–82.

30. Hlavaty T, Huorka M, Koller T, et al. Colorectal cancer screening in patients with ulcerative and Crohn's colitis with use of colonoscopy, chromoendoscopy and confocal endomicroscopy. Eur J Gastroenterol Hepatol 2011;23:680–9.

31. Hurlstone DP, Sanders DS, Lobo AJ, et al. Indigo carmine-assisted high-magnification chromoscopic colonoscopy for the detection and characterisation of intraepithelial neoplasia in ulcerative colitis: a prospective evaluation. Endoscopy 2005;37:1186–92.

32. Gunther U, Kusch D, Heller F, et al. Surveillance colonoscopy in patients with inflammatory bowel disease: comparison of random biopsy vs. targeted biopsy protocols. Int J Colorectal Dis 2011;26:667–72.

33. van den Broek FJ, van Es JA, van Eeden S, et al. Pilot study of probe-based confocal laser endomicroscopy during colonoscopic surveillance of patients with longstanding ulcerative colitis. Endoscopy 2011;43:116–22.

34. Su P, Liu Y, Lin S, et al. Efficacy of confocal laser endomicroscopy for discriminating colorectal neoplasms from non-neoplasms: a systematic review and meta-analysis. Colorectal Dis 2013;15:e1–12.

35. Wanders LK, Kuiper T, Kiesslich R, et al. Limited applicability of chromoendoscopy-guided confocal laser endomicroscopy as daily-practice surveillance strategy in Crohn's disease. Gastrointest Endosc 2015;83:966–71.

36. Heif M, Yen RD, Shah RJ. ERCP with probe-based confocal laser endomicroscopy for the evaluation of dominant biliary stenoses in primary sclerosing cholangitis patients. Dig Dis Sci 2013;58:2068–74.

37. Hsiung PL, Hardy J, Friedland S, et al. Detection of colonic dysplasia in vivo using a targeted heptapeptide and confocal microendoscopy. Nat Med 2008;14:454–8.

38. Goetz M, Ziebart A, Foersch S, et al. In vivo molecular imaging of colorectal cancer with confocal endomicroscopy by targeting epidermal growth factor receptor. Gastroenterology 2010;138:435–46.

39. Goetz M, Hoetker MS, Diken M, et al. In vivo molecular imaging with cetuximab, an anti-EGFR antibody, for prediction of response in xenograft models of human colorectal cancer. Endoscopy 2013;45:469–77.

40. Schmidt C, Lautenschlaeger C, Collnot EM, et al. Nano- and microscaled particles for drug targeting to inflamed intestinal mucosa: a first in vivo study in human patients. J Control Release 2013;165:139–45.

41. Atreya R, Neumann H, Neufert C, et al. In vivo imaging using fluorescent antibodies to tumor necrosis factor predicts therapeutic response in Crohn's disease. Nat Med 2014;20:313–8.

42. Neumann H, Vieth M, Atreya R, et al. Prospective evaluation of the learning curve of confocal laser endomicroscopy in patients with IBD. Histol Histopathol 2011;26:867–72.

The Evaluation of Postoperative Patients with Ulcerative Colitis

Bo Shen, MD

KEYWORDS

- Crohn's disease • Endoscopy • Ileal pouch • Pouchitis • Pouchoscopy
- Restorative proctocolectomy • Ulcerative colitis • Ileoscopy

KEY POINTS

- Restorative proctocolectomy with ileal pouch-anal anastomosis has become the standard surgical treatment modality for patients with ulcerative colitis or familial adenomatous polyposis who require colectomy.
- Normally staged pouch surgery is performed. The classic 2-stage restorative proctocolectomy involves (1) total proctocolectomy, the creation of a J or S pouch with anastomosis to a short rectal stump, and loop ileostomy and (2) closure of loop ileostomy.
- In patients with severe colitis and strong immunosuppression, a 3-stage surgery is advocated, which consists of (1) subtotal colectomy and end ileostomy; (2) ileal pouch construction and anastomosis, loop ileostomy; and (3) closure of the loop ileostomy.
- Endoscopy plays an important role in postoperative monitoring of disease status and delivery of therapy, if necessary.
- Ileal pouch surgery significantly alters bowel anatomy, with new organ structures being created.
- Endoscopy of the altered bowel includes the evaluation of end ileostomy, Hartmann pouch or diverted rectum, loop ileostomy, diverted pouch, and pouchoscopy.
- Each segment of the bowel has unique landmarks. It is important for endoscopists to be familiar with those landmarks and recognize the status of healthy and diseased.

INTRODUCTION

The last 2 decades have witnessed a great progress in medical therapy for inflammatory bowel disease (IBD), including Crohn's disease (CD) and ulcerative colitis (UC). The availability and wide use of anti–tumor necrosis factor (TNF) and anti-integrin biological agents have revolutionized the management of IBD. However,

Disclosure: The author has received honoraria from Abbvie and Janssen; research grant from Aptalis; and education grant from Abbvie and Janssen.
The Interventional IBD (i-IBD) Unit-Desk A31, Digestive Disease and Surgery Institute, The Cleveland Clinic Foundation, 9500 Euclid Avenue, Cleveland, OH 44195, USA
E-mail address: shenb@ccf.org

approximately 20% to 30% of patients with UC will eventually need colectomy for medically refractory disease or colitis-associated neoplasia. Restorative proctocolectomy (RTC) with ileal pouch-anal anastomosis (IPAA) is the surgical treatment of choice for patients with UC who require colectomy. RTC and IPAA are technically challenging procedures with a risk for the development of various forms of complications. In addition, inflammatory and even neoplastic conditions can develop after colectomy. In most patients, their underlying IBD is still not considered as being cured after RPC and IPAA.

One-stage RPC and IPAA are rarely offered to patients. The standard 2-stage RPC involves (1) total proctocolectomy (TPC), the creation of a J or S pouch with anastomosis to rectal stump, and loop ileostomy (LI) and (2) closure of LI. In patients with severe colitis and strong immunosuppression, a 3-stage surgery is advocated, which consists of (1) subtotal colectomy (STC) leaving a diverted rectum, also named Hartmann pouch, and end ileostomy (EI); (2) ileal pouch construction and anastomosis and LI; and (3) closure of LI. The staged procedures create de novo anatomic structures, including Hartmann pouch, EI, LI, diverted pouch, and connected pouch. Various disease conditions can occur in those segments of the bowel. Anatomic classification of surgery-altered bowel in UC is listed in **Table 1**.

Proctoscopy for Hartmann Pouch

In patients with severe or fulminant colitis, STC, rather than TPC, should be performed. With the extensive immunosuppressive agents, such as corticosteroids[1] and anti-TNF agents, there have been concerns for the increased risk for postoperative infectious complications.[2,3] The first of the 3-stage RPC and IPAA involves STC, EI, and Hartmann pouch reduce the risk for postoperative infectious complications. The length of a Hartmann pouch can be 10 to 25 cm, depending on the degree of the concern of stump leak. For patients with severe colitis and a significant concern of stump leak, surgeons temporarily leave a long rectal stump, which is connected to the abdominal fascia, to reduce the risk for intrapelvic abscess in case stump leaks.

Diversion proctitis can develop, largely because of the lack of nutrients from luminal bacteria to the rectal mucosa. Patients may present with pelvic discomfort and pain, urgency, and mucous or bloody discharge. On endoscopy, there can be extremely friable mucosa, even with minimum air insufflation, edema, erythema, ulcers,

Table 1
Bowel anatomy after colectomy for ulcerative colitis

Name	Configuration	Duration of Creation	Purpose of Creation
Ileostomy	End ileostomy	Temporary	Primary (for setting stage for subsequent pouch surgery)
		Permanent	Primary (for those with colectomy without intention for having an ileal pouch)
			Secondary (due to failed pouch)
	Loop ileostomy	Temporary	Setup for subsequent initial pouch construction or pouch revision surgery
Pouch	Hartmann pouch	Temporary	Equivalent to diverted rectum
	Diverted pouch		Primary (set-up stage for initial construction or pouch revision)
		Permanent	Secondary (due to pouch failure with permanent fecal diversion)
	Connected pouch	Permanent	Functioned pouch

nodularity, and exudates (**Fig. 1**A). Histology of diversion proctitis is characterized by the presence of diffuse lymphoid hyperplasia.

In non-IBD patients, the best treatment option for diversion proctitis is the restoration of fecal continuity. In patients for undergoing for RPC and IPAA, Hartmann pouch or diversion pouchitis is a temporary measure. Symptomatic patients may be treated with topical mesalamine, corticosteroids, or short-chain fatty enema.

Ileoscopy Via Stoma for End Ileostomy

In patients with UC with RPC and IPAA, EI is usually created in the following 2 settings: (1) as an initial *temporary* part of a 3-stage pouch surgery, with an intention to convert LI during pouch construction or (2) as a *permanent* diversion in patients who elect not to have a pouch after TPC (the primary EI) or in those with a failed pouch due to various mechanical, inflammatory, or neoplastic complications (the secondary EI).

Ileoscopy via stoma for patients with a temporary EI is needed before pouch construction and conversion of EI to LI for the purpose of ruling out CD of the small bowel, although inflammation and/or ulcers are extremely rare in patients with UC undergoing colectomy. Mucosal biopsy is still needed. In rare occasions, postcolectomy enteritis syndrome can occur soon after colectomy in patients with the primary EI and a preoperative diagnosis of UC. The patients with this disease entity may present with significant increased ileostomy output, dehydration, and malnutrition. On endoscopy, this syndrome is characterized with diffuse mucosal inflammation, which is different from the segmental inflammation in CD.

Pouch failure is defined as permanent fecal diversion with the secondary EI, pouch excision, or pouch revision. Patients with permanent secondary EI due to pouch failure should be closely monitored for disease recurrence, particularly CD-associated inflammation, ulcers, and stricture.[4]

Ileoscopy Via Stoma for Loop Ileostomy

In most cases, LI is created for a temporary purpose with an intention of anticipated closure. Despite the difficulty in the management of stoma, with a higher risk for stomal or peristomal complications than EI, it offers an easier closure procedure than the EI. In staged pouch surgery, LI is created to allow for the maturation of the anastomosis and other sutures of a newly constructed pouch. LI is occasionally performed as a part of treatment of mechanical or inflammatory complications of the pouch to cool down the disease by fecal diversion. In both cases, ileoscopy via stoma to the

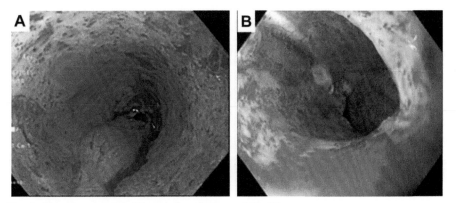

Fig. 1. Diversion proctitis (*A*) and diversion pouchitis (*B*).

afferent limb of LI is needed for all patients before undergoing LI closure to rule out CD. Inflammation, ulcers, or strictures in the distal bowel segment through the abdominal wall are not necessarily CD and may result from ischemia.

Pouchoscopy for Diverted Pouch

In the staged pouch surgery, patients typically carry a diverted pouch for 3 to 6 months before restoration of fecal continuity. Because of the lacking nutrients from luminal bacteria, diversion pouchitis is common, which is characterized by erythema, edema, friability, erosions, and ulcers (see **Fig. 1**B).

Permanent fecal diversion with ileostomy and pouch in situ is routinely performed in patients with pouch failure. It has been controversial in the management of diverted pouch in long-term, excision of the failed pouch versus keep the pouch in situ. The excision of the pouch is a technically demanding surgery, involving removal of pouch as well as internal and external anal sphincter muscles. Its associated complications include stump leak, sinus, and abscess. Occasionally small bowel obstruction can occur due to the location of stoma and the downward displacement of the space of pouch body with the distal small bowel. On the other hand, keeping the pouch in situ can also have issues, particularly diversion pouchitis, distal pouch stricture, and the risk for neoplasia. Patients with diversion pouchitis can present with excessive discharge of mucus and/or bloody material, urgency, incontinence, abdominal cramps. Long-term diversion increases the risk for the development of the distal pouch or anastomotic stricture. A severe stricture can result in a completely sealed pouch outlet with accumulation of large quantity of liquid luminal contents or even bezoar, which can lead to abdominal and pelvic discomfort and pain (**Fig. 2**). As the mucosa is often friable, endoscopy for the diverted pouch should be carefully performed, with a minimum air insufflation and avoidance of deep biopsy. The stricture can be treated with endoscopic balloon dilation or endoscopic needle knife stricturotomy. The latter with a targeted spot and depth of treatment seems to be less invasive and more effective.

There are no published data on the prevalence or incidence of neoplasia of diverted pouch, anal transitional zone (ATZ) or cuff in patients with UC or FAP. Because the prognosis of pouch cancer is poor,[5] this author recommends that patients at high risk, such as those with a precolectomy diagnosis of colon neoplasia or FAP, should have a yearly pouchoscopy with biopsy, even in those with mucosectomy during IPAA surgery. Special attention should be paid to the ATZ and cuff.

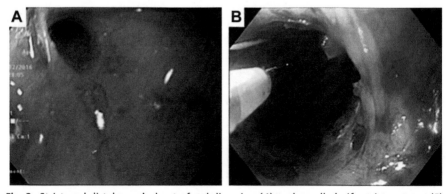

Fig. 2. Strictured distal pouch due to fecal diversion (A) and needle knife stricturotomy (B).

Pouchoscopy for Connected Pouch

The purpose of pouchoscopy here are severalfold: (1) diagnosis of mechanical and inflammatory complications of the pouch, (2) surveillance for neoplasia, and (3) delivery of endoscopic therapy. The common mechanical complications of IPAA surgery can roughly be divided into 2 categories: (1) obstruction and (2) leak. The obstructive disease conditions include (1) strictures at the anastomosis, pouch body, inlet, and afferent limb and LI site; (2) angulation of bowel loop, such as afferent limb and efferent limb syndromes; and (3) twisted pouch and pouch prolapse. The leak conditions of the pouch include acute and chronic complications, including acute anastomotic leak with or without abscess or pelvic sepsis and chronic leak with sinus. The common locations of the leak are the tip of the J and anastomosis. In the latter condition, there can be presacral sinus posteriorly and pouch vaginal fistula anterior. This author recommends that in patients with suspected surgery-associated mechanical complications, abdominal/pelvic imaging is needed to provide the roadmap for the subsequent diagnostic and/or therapeutic pouchoscopy. The mechanical complications of the pouch, which may be amenable for endoscopic therapy, include strictures (treated with endoscopic balloon dilation or needle knife stricturotomy), presacral sinus (treated with needle knife sinusotomy), and the leak at the tip of the J (treated with over-the-scope clipping system).

The main inflammatory complications of the IPAA are pouchitis, CD of the pouch (CDP), and cuffitis. Endoscopy is the most important diagnostic modality for those disorders. The endoscopy should carefully examine all segments and landmarks of IPAA, including LI site, afferent limb, pouch inlet, tip of the J, pouch body, and ATZ or cuff, along with perianal regions. The distribution and severity of inflammation and the location of stricture or fistula should be carefully documented. The Pouchitis Disease Activity Index with its endoscopy subscore has been used for the assessment of the degree of inflammation in pouchitis,[6] which is also extrapolated into CDP[7] or cuffitis.[8]

It is thought that the cause and pathogenesis of pouchitis are related to dysbiosis and dysregulated mucosal immunity. The genetic factors and surgery-associated ischemia may play a role in a subset of patients. Pouchitis may be classified into 3 main categories based on etiopathogenesis: (1) microbiota-associated pouchitis, (2) immune-mediated pouchitis, and (3) ischemia-associated pouchitis. Endoscopic features, particularly the distribution pattern of inflammation, may provide clues for the cause of pouchitis.[9] Inflammation of dysbiosis-associated pouchitis is usually limited to the pouch body, sparing the afferent limb and cuff. Inflammation of immune-mediated pouchitis usually involves both the pouch body and afferent limb and in some cases the cuff. The classic example of immune-mediated pouchitis is primary sclerosing cholangitis (PSC)-associated pouchitis/enteritis with the presence of a long segment of enteritis above the pouch inlet in addition to diffuse pouch inflammation. Ischemic pouchitis is presented with asymmetric distribution of inflammation; and inflammation may only involve the afferent limb side of the pouch body, the distal pouch body only, or the suture line only[10] (**Fig. 3**A–C). For pouchitis, endoscopic biopsy is needed, not for grading inflammation, rather, for the assessment of features of pyloric gland metaplasia (indicating chronic mucosa injury), mucosal hemorrhage, cytomegalovirus, granulomas, and neoplasia.

CD or a CD-like condition can develop after IPAA for patients with a preoperative diagnosis of UC or indeterminate colitis.[11] There are a wide range of clinical presentations, endoscopic and histologic features, and prognoses in CDP. Based on the clinical behavior, CDP is categorized into (1) inflammatory, (2) stricturing, and (3) fistulizing

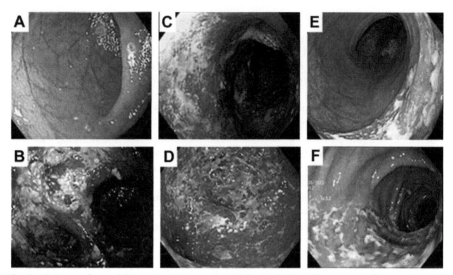

Fig. 3. Pattern of pouchitis: microbiota-associated pouchitis with normal afferent limb (*A*) and inflammation of pouch body (*B*); immune-mediated pouchitis with diffuse inflammation in both afferent limb (*C*) and pouch body (*D*); and ischemic pouchitis with inflammation only at the distal pouch (*E*) or afferent limb of pouch body (*F*) and a sharp demarcation between inflamed and noninflamed portions.

phenotypes (**Fig. 4**).[12] Pouch endoscopy is the most important diagnostic modality for the diagnosis and management of CDP. The disease process in CDP is not limited to the pouch body. In fact, it can involve any parts of the gastrointestinal track, including the stomach, proximal and distal small bowel, and cuff. A careful evaluation of the pattern and distribution of mucosal ulceration and inflammation on pouchoscopy is needed. Endoscopic features of CDP include discrete or segmental small and large ulcers, nodularity, exudate, and/or inflammatory pseudopolyps in the pouch body, afferent limb, cuff, or ATZ. Prepouch ileitis may be present in patients with pouchitis, which does not necessarily indicate CD.

CDP may present with a stricturing phenotype. The stricture can occur at the anastomosis, pouch body, inlet, ileostomy site, and afferent limb or even the upper gastrointestinal track. Those strictures can also occur in patients with the use of nonsteroidal

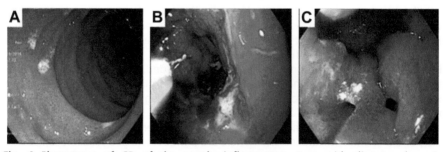

Fig. 4. Phenotypes of CD of the pouch: inflammatory type with discrete ulcers in the afferent limb (*A*), stricturing type with needle knife stricturotomy (*B*), and fistulizing type (*C*).

antiinflammatory drugs (NSAIDs). In addition, ischemia-related injury can mimic CDP and NSAID-induced injury. Avoidance of NSAIDs and a diagnostic trial of biologics may help differentiate the 3 disease entities from each other.[13]

Fistulizing CDP is one of the most challenging entities to diagnose and manage. In addition to fistulizing CDP, surgery-associated ischemia, iatrogenic injury, and cryptoglandular abscess can also occur. There can be a pouch-vaginal fistula, perianal fistula, and enterocutaneous fistula. Enterocutaneous fistula often results from a leak at the tip of the J leak. It is important to identify the fistula opening from the pouch side and delineate the length and configuration of fistula. This can be achieved by the use of an endoscopic guidewire or spray of hydrogen peroxide, methylene blue, or povidone-iodine (Betadine). MRI of the pelvis or examination under general anesthesia in the operating room may help confirm the diagnosis. The presence of the following features suggests the diagnosis of CDP: (1) the presence of fistula opening in the mid anal canal, outside of the anastomosis, dentate line, or the tip of the J; (2) inflammation around the fistula opening; (3) complex fistula, that is, multiple fistulae or branched fistula; (4) fistula and inflammation and ulcers at separate locations of the pouch; and (5) the development of fistula more than 12 months after ileostomy closure. The presence of nonmucinous, noncaseating granulomas on histology normally suggests a diagnosis of CDP. Unfortunately, only 10% of patients with known CDP had granulomas on mucosal biopsy. Endoscopists should resist the temptation to take mucosal biopsy from the normal or ulcerated suture line, in order to avoid the confusion from foreign-body granulomas or pseudogranulomas.

Cuffitis has been considered as the remnant UC. However, other disorders can also cause pouch inflammation, such as ischemia, prolapse, CD, or neoplasia[8,14] (**Fig. 5**).

Patients with UC with RPC and IPAA still carry some risk for pouch neoplasia. Although dysplasia may occur in both pouch body and cuff or ATZ, cancerous lesions have been almost exclusively detected at the cuff or ATZ.[15,16] The main risk factors for pouch neoplasia is a precolectomy diagnosis of colon or rectal neoplasia.[14,15] Yearly surveillance pouchoscopy is recommended for patients with the risk factor. Other potential risk factors are the presence of PSC, family history of colon cancer, chronic pouchitis, and chronic cuffitis. Patients with those risk factors may undergo surveillance pouchoscopy every 1 to 3 years. For those without any of the risk factors, surveillance pouchoscopy may be performed every 3 years after the diagnosis of UC for more than 10 years.[17] During the surveillance biopsy, segmental biopsy of the pouch body and cuff or ATZ is taken, with 3 to 4 pieces for each location. Not all pouch neoplasia have endoscopically visible lesions.[14] Chromoendoscopy may help to highlight the neoplastic lesion.

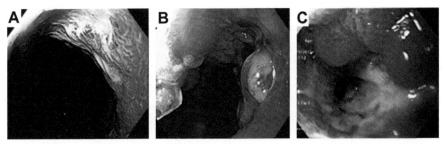

Fig. 5. Pattern of cuffitis: classic cuffitis, representing a remnant form of UC (*A*), prolapse-associated cuffitis (*B*), and CD-related cuffitis (*C*).

SUMMARY

Endoscopy plays a key role for surgical planning, disease monitoring, diagnosis, differential diagnosis, neoplasia surveillance, and delivery of therapy at different stages of RPC and IPAA. Endoscopy is the most reliable modality in grading mucosal inflammation.

REFERENCES

1. Ferrante M, D'Hoore A, Vermeire S, et al. Corticosteroids but not infliximab increase short-term postoperative infectious complications in patients with ulcerative colitis. Inflamm Bowel Dis 2009;15:1062–70.
2. Gu J, Remzi FH, Shen B, et al. Operative strategy modifies risk of pouch-related outcomes in patients with ulcerative colitis on preoperative anti-tumor necrosis factor-α therapy. Dis Colon Rectum 2013;56:1243–52.
3. Mor IJ, Vogel JD, da Luz Moreira A, et al. Infliximab in ulcerative colitis is associated with an increased risk of postoperative complications after restorative proctocolectomy. Dis Colon Rectum 2008;51:1202–7 [discussion: 1207–10].
4. Du P, Sun C, Ashburn J, et al. Risk factors for Crohn's disease of the neo-small intestine in ulcerative colitis patients with total proctocolectomy and primary or secondary ileostomies. J Crohns Colitis 2015;9:170–6.
5. Wu XR, Remzi FH, Liu XL, et al. Disease course and management strategy of pouch neoplasia in patients with underlying inflammatory bowel diseases. Inflamm Bowel Dis 2014;20:2073–82.
6. Sandborn WJ, Tremaine WJ, Batts KP, et al. Pouchitis after ileal pouch-anal anastomosis: a Pouchitis Disease Activity Index. Mayo Clin Proc 1994;69:409–15.
7. Shen B, Fazio VW, Remzi FH, et al. Clinical features and quality of life in patients with different phenotypes of Crohn's disease of the ileal pouch. Dis Colon Rectum 2007;50:1450–9.
8. Wu B, Lian L, Li Y, et al. Clinical course of cuffitis in ulcerative colitis patients with restorative proctocolectomy and ileal pouch-anal anastomoses. Inflamm Bowel Dis 2013;19:404–10.
9. Shen B. Problems after restorative proctocolectomy: assessment and therapy. Curr Opin Gastroenterol 2016;32:49–54.
10. Shen B, Plesec TP, Remer E, et al. Asymmetric inflammation of ileal pouch: a sign for ischemic pouchitis? Inflamm Bowel Dis 2010;16:836–46.
11. Melton GB, Fazio VW, Kiran RP, et al. Long-term outcomes with ileal pouch-anal anastomosis and Crohn's disease: pouch retention and implications of delayed diagnosis. Ann Surg 2008;248:608–16.
12. Shen B, Fazio VW, Remzi FH, et al. Risk factors for clinical phenotypes of Crohn's disease of the pouch. Am J Gastroenterol 2006;101:2760–8.
13. Shen B, Fazio VW, Bennett AE, et al. Effect of withdrawal of non-steroidal anti-inflammatory drug use in patients with the ileal pouch. Dig Dis Sci 2007;52:3321–8.
14. Shen B, Liu X. De novo collagenous cuffitis. Inflamm Bowel Dis 2011;17:1249–50.
15. Kariv R, Remzi FH, Lian L, et al. Preoperative colorectal neoplasia increases risk for pouch neoplasia in patients with restorative proctocolectomy. Gastroenterology 2010;139:806–12.
16. Derikx LA, Kievit W, Drenth JP, et al, Dutch Initiative on Crohn and Colitis. Prior colorectal neoplasia is associated with increased risk of ileoanal pouch

neoplasia in patients with inflammatory bowel disease. Gastroenterology 2014; 146:119–28.

17. Liu ZX, Kiran RP, Bennett AE, et al. Diagnosis and management of dysplasia and cancer of the ileal pouch in patients with underlying inflammatory bowel disease. Cancer 2011;117:3081–92.

Endoscopic Evaluation and Management of the Postoperative Crohn's Disease Patient

Jana G. Hashash, MD, MSc[a], David G. Binion, MD, AGAF[b],*

KEYWORDS

- Crohn's disease • Side-to-side anastomosis • End-to-end anastomosis
- End-to-side anastomosis • Rutgeerts endoscopic score • Anastomotic stricture
- Balloon dilatation

KEY POINTS

- A majority of Crohn's disease (CD) patients require surgery with ileocecal resection being the most common procedure.
- CD anastomotic recurrence can be quantified using Rutgeerts endoscopic score within 1 year of surgery, which carries prognostic significance and can guide therapy.
- The 4 most common anastomotic configurations include end-to-end, end-to-side, anti-peristaltic side-to-side, and isoperistaltic side-to-side reconstructions.
- Anastomotic reconstruction after ileocecal resection varies with antiperistaltic, side-to-side anastomosis surpassing end-to-end anastomosis at the present time.
- CD anastomotic recurrence in the antiperistaltic side-to-side anastomosis occurs at the inlet, which is typically seen on retroflex view.

INTRODUCTION

Approximately 70% of patients with CD undergo surgical resection for the treatment of medically refractory disease or its complications during their lifetime. The sickest cohort of CD patients experiences rapid postoperative relapse at the anastomotic

Disclosure Statement: Dr J.G. Hashash: Nothing to disclose. Dr D.G. Binion has received consulting honoraria from Janssen Biotech and UCB Pharma as well as grant support from Janssen Biotech, UCB Pharma, and Merck.
[a] Division of Gastroenterology, Hepatology and Nutrition, UPMC-Presbyterian Hospital, University of Pittsburgh School of Medicine, 200 Lothrop Street, Mezzanine Level C Wing PUH, Pittsburgh, PA 15213, USA; [b] Division of Gastroenterology, Hepatology and Nutrition, Clinical and Translational Science, UPMC-Presbyterian Hospital, University of Pittsburgh School of Medicine, 200 Lothrop Street, Mezzanine Level C Wing PUH, Pittsburgh, PA 15213, USA
* Corresponding author.
E-mail address: binion@pitt.edu

Gastrointest Endoscopy Clin N Am 26 (2016) 679–692
http://dx.doi.org/10.1016/j.giec.2016.06.003
1052-5157/16/$ – see front matter © 2016 Elsevier Inc. All rights reserved.

giendo.theclinics.com

site, which can lead to repeated surgeries. A majority of CD patients have a reconstruction of the intestine after surgery, where a surgical anastomosis connects the upstream and downstream segments of bowel, whereas other patients require an ostomy. Over the past 2 decades, the types of surgical anastomoses used in CD reconstruction have changed, where end-to-side and end-to-end anastomoses have been surpassed by the more rapidly created side-to-side anastomoses (antiperistaltic orientation and isoperistaltic orientation). Although high-definition white light endoscopes have allowed for enhanced assessment of the postoperative mucosal surface, there is limited information at this time that helps inform and guide gastroenterologists regarding endoscopic assessment of surgically altered anatomy, particularly in regard to the different types of anastomoses. This article provides a comprehensive review of the timing and purpose of endoscopic evaluation in postoperative CD patients and provides pragmatic information regarding interpretation of endoscopic findings at the different types of surgical anastomoses after ileocecal resection.

SURGERY AND CROHN'S DISEASE: ASSESSING POSTOPERATIVE CROHN'S DISEASE RECURRENCE

Ileocecal resection is the hallmark operation for CD, dating back to the original description of the disease in 1932, where 14 patients with terminal ileal strictures underwent resection after radiographic characterization.[1] This historical perspective is relevant today, because a majority of CD patients require surgery, but radiographic studies have now been complemented with colonoscopy and direct mucosal assessment of the preoperative and postoperative mucosa. The importance of endoscopic assessment of postoperative CD patients stems directly from the fact that there are different patterns of CD recurrence and this heterogeneous natural history may be linked to personalized approaches tailored to maintain the surgically induced clinical remission. Endoscopy offers an opportunity to not only visualize the site of surgery but also allow for characterization of the early return of mucosal ulceration, not yet radiographically apparent, which carries important prognostic significance. Furthermore, mucosal pinch biopsies at the level of the anastomosis give additional information that can help personalize therapeutic intervention. Lastly, in certain situations, an anastomotic stricture may form and endoscopically guided pneumatic balloon dilatation with or without intralesional steroid injection can be attempted to re-establish luminal patency. The ability to endoscopically assess the surgical anastomosis and the neoterminal ileum in the postoperative time period for diagnostic, prognostic, and therapeutic purposes is essential for improving CD clinical outcomes.

ENDOSCOPIC ASSESSMENT OF THE CROHN'S DISEASE ANASTOMOSIS: GAUGING POSTOPERATIVE RECURRENCE AND TAILORING THERAPY

The ability to effectively gauge CD activity at the postoperative neoterminal ileum is dependent on a structured assessment where objective endoscopic features are linked to a predictable natural history over the ensuing years. The postoperative CD patient provides the best opportunity to standardize an endoscopic assessment score, because the neoterminal ileum is essentially free of disease after surgical reconstruction, and the return of CD lesions over a known time (eg, the date of surgery) offers an opportunity to characterize disease trajectories. The development of a postoperative neoterminal ileal score, which was associated with clinical CD recurrence, was achieved by Rutgeerts and colleagues[2] in Leuven, Belgium, in the early 1990s. Using a cohort of 89 postoperative CD patients, these investigators developed an endoscopic scoring system to grade the severity of mucosal ulceration at the neoterminal ileum 1 year after resection and were able to associate patterns of ulceration with subsequent clinical recurrence over the next 6 years.[2] The Rutgeerts endoscopic scoring system grades the severity of recurrent CD in the postoperative patient by focusing on the mucosa of the ileocolonic anastomosis and the neoterminal ileum, just proximal to the anastomosis. Scores range from an ileal endoscopic score of i0 to i4, the latter score indicative of more severe endoscopic recurrence (the majority of neoterminal ileal mucosa is ulcerated). The score i0 indicates an endoscopically normal neoterminal ileum, whereas the emergence of scattered aphthous ulcers (<5 ulcers) is classified as a Rutgeerts i1 score. More than 5 aphthous ulcers in the neoterminal ileum is defined as a Rutgeerts i2 score. Deeper, discrete stellate ulcers constitute a Rutgeerts i3 score (ulcers involve <50% of the lumen), and the most severe recurrence, Rutgeerts i4 score, demonstrates linear ulcers encompassing more than 50% of the lumen, representing the most significant recurrence. **Table 1** defines the different endoscopic scores of the Rutgeerts score and **Fig. 1** displays the corresponding endoscopic images of different recurrence scores at the neoterminal ileum.

Patients with an ileal Rutgeerts score of i0 or i1 are considered in endoscopic remission in the postoperative time period. The prognostic component of the score suggests that a majority of these individuals do not require medical therapy, because they have a low probability of developing clinical recurrence of their CD over the ensuing years.[2] One of the most important insights that arose from the development of the Rutgeerts score was the understanding that a majority of postoperative CD patients remain asymptomatic for up to 3 years after their surgery/reanastomosis, which is irrespective of early endoscopic features seen at the anastomosis 1 year after surgery. Although demonstrating objective evidence of CD recurrence at the anastomosis, a majority of postoperative CD patients with more severe endoscopic recurrence (i4) 1 year after surgery experience clinical relapse (70% by 1 year after surgery).[2] CD patients with i3 recurrence 1 year after surgery have a 1-year clinical recurrence rate of 30% and a 50% recurrence rate by year 4.[2] This identification of silent endoscopic recurrence that portends a clinical relapse in the ensuing years highlighted the importance of assessing and documenting objective evidence of recurrence in the year after surgery. Patients with aggressive return of mucosal lesions seen on endoscopy essentially declared themselves appropriate candidates for postoperative treatment, with immunomodulator and/or biologic agents, prior to the return of significant damaging disease, which might otherwise be less responsive to therapy.

Although the Rutgeerts score was never validated for postoperative CD treatment trials, the score has been used to define endoscopic recurrence and has been used in several studies assessing the efficacy of preventing CD recurrence in the

Table 1		
Definition of Rutgeerts postoperative endoscopic ileal scores		
Endoscopic Score	**Definition**	
i0	No lesions	
i1	≤5 Aphthous lesions	
i2	>5 Aphthous lesions with normal mucosa between the lesions or skip areas of larger lesions or lesions confined to the ileocolonic anastomosis	
i3	Diffuse aphthous ileitis with diffusely inflamed mucosa	
i4	Diffuse inflammation with already larger ulcers, nodules, and/or narrowing	

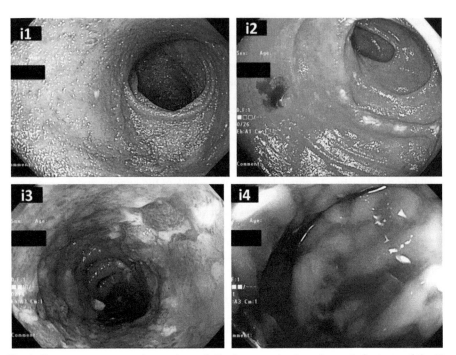

Fig. 1. Rutgeerts postoperative endoscopic ileal scores; classic endoscopic features of the i0, i1, i2, i3, and i4 scores are demonstrated.

postoperative time period. In a majority of studies, clinical recurrence remained the primary endpoint whereas patterns of endoscopic recurrence were designated secondary endpoints. In a recent study by De Cruz et al., the authors developed and prospectively validated a new postoperative endoscopic index of severity (POCER Index) by assessing number (0, $\leq$2, >2), size (1-5mm vs $\geq$6mm), depth (superficial vs deep), and circumferential extent (<25% vs $\geq$25%) of anastomotic ulcers. Detection of deep ulcers and more extensive anastomotic ulceration ($\geq$25%) at a 6 month post-operative time period were highly associated with significant endoscopic recurrence (Rutgeerts ileal score i$\geq$2) at an 18 month post-operative time period. This simplified endoscopic staging may ultimately prove useful in stratifying post-operative CD patients to receive immunomodulator and/or biologic therapy following surgery.[3]

Early attempts to delay postoperative recurrence of CD demonstrated marginal benefit of 5 aminosalicylic agents, antibiotics, and purine analog agents.[4–11] More significant results were demonstrated with the use of postoperative biologic agents, which showed significant benefit regarding the prevention of CD endoscopic recurrence.[12–20]

In 2015 and 2016, 2 multicenter clinical trials were published, which used the Rutgeerts score as a key component in a step-up approach for managing postoperative CD as well as assessing the efficacy of postoperative biologic therapy. In the POCER (Post-Operative Crohn's Endoscopic Recurrence) trial, postoperative CD patients underwent endoscopic assessment and, based on the patterns of recurrence, were stratified to receive immunomodulators and/or biologic agents.[21] In the PREVENT (Infliximab for Prevention of Recurrence of Post-Surgical Crohn's Disease Following Ileocolonic Resection: a Randomized, Placebo-Controlled Study) trial, which randomized patients to receive infliximab versus placebo infusions in the postoperative time period, there was a significant decrease in patterns of endoscopic recurrence at 18 months.[22] Unfortunately, the primary end point of the trial was a composite score composed of both clinical symptoms and endoscopic recurrence, which was not met in interim analysis. As a result, the trial was halted prematurely due to the failure to achieve a predesignated clinical recurrence prevention endpoint. The rates of endoscopic recurrence of CD were cut in half, however, in the patients who received active therapy.

PRACTICAL GUIDANCE: ENDOSCOPIC EVALUATION GUIDES MANAGEMENT OF POSTOPERATIVE CROHN'S DISEASE

The growing consensus from published evidence suggests that endoscopic evaluation of the colonic and ileal mucosa helps guide CD medical therapy in the postoperative setting. Although there are no official guidelines, the authors recommend that postoperative CD patients undergo an ileocolonoscopy 6 to 12 months after their intestinal resection to evaluate the anastomosis and the neoterminal ileum just proximal to the anastomosis.[23,24] The reproducible patterns of CD recurrence make this targeted assessment very high yield in terms of prognostication and stratification for further medical therapy, because the intestine just proximal to the anastomosis has the highest likelihood for CD recurrence.

Currently there are 2 strategies for approaching postoperative CD; the first is watchful waiting and only starting patients with high risk for recurrence on a prophylactic medication, whereas the other strategy (and the authors' preference) is to start high-risk and moderate-risk patients on a prophylactic medication.[23] At 6 to 12 months postoperatively, patients undergo a colonoscopy to evaluate for postoperative CD recurrence, and, depending on the presence of endoscopic lesions (Rutgeerts ileal score > i2), medical management is modified, either medication escalated or changed.

Given the emergence of data suggesting benefit of immunosuppressive and/or biologic therapy when used in the early postoperative time period, it is recommended that patients who undergo ileocecectomy with an anastomosis have an ileocolonoscopy as early as 6 to 12 months postoperatively. The purpose of this early and typically asymptomatic endoscopic assessment is to evaluate for early postoperative recurrence of CD to optimize medical therapy in a timely fashion, prior to the recurrence of significant inflammation and irreversible damage and tissue remodeling. This is particularly true for CD patients who choose to go on no form of postoperative medical therapy after resection and reanastomosis.

POSTOPERATIVE SURGICAL ANATOMY IN CROHN'S DISEASE: PRAGMATIC APPROACH TO ENDOSCOPIC ASSESSMENT OF THE ANASTOMOTIC CONFIGURATION

As discussed previously, the most common CD surgery is an ileocecal resection with ileocolonic anastomosis. The type of reconstruction after ileocecal resection varies, however, with essentially 4 different configurations comprising the majority of anastomoses. At present, the American Society of Colon and Rectal Surgeons does not recommend one type of surgical anastomosis over another, because the best prospective multicenter trial data assessing end-to-end versus side-to-side anastomoses did not demonstrate superior or inferior outcomes, which included operative complications, leaks, and patterns of CD recurrence at 1 year.[25] Thus, society recommendations have left the choice of anastomotic configuration to the discretion of the treating surgeon. More recent prospective, observational data generated by the Inflammatory Bowel Disease Center at the University of Pittsburgh Medical Center (UPMC) suggest, however, that not all anastomotic configurations are equal when considering

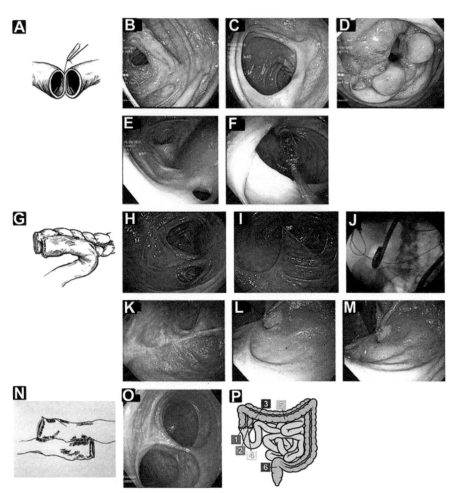

Fig. 2. Endoscopic interpretation of anastomotic configuration after ileocecal resection in CD. (*A–E*) End-to-end anastomosis. Endoscopic appearance of an end-to-end ileocolonic anastomosis. Note that the lumen continues in a straight orientation. Mucosal assessment of the vascular pattern varies between the colonic and ileal segments. Given the tubelike configuration of this type of anastomosis, endoscopic assessment in the postoperative time period is readily achieved. (*D*) Endoscopic appearance of a strictured end-to-end ileocolonic anastomosis in CD demonstrates an edematous, congested mucosa, which may not allow for intubation. Anchoring sutures, often bile stained, provide orientation regarding the anastomosis. This patient developed obstructive symptoms postoperatively and was able to benefit from TTS endoscopic balloon dilatation. (*E, F*) End-to-side anastomosis. (*E*) End-to-side ileocolonic anastomosis with stricture that was dilated using TTS balloon. The stapled off native ileocolonic valve is in the distance and an anastomosis into the side wall is evident. The web stricture did not initially allow for intubation by the adult colonoscope. (*F*) TTS balloon was deployed across the stricture, which was dilated successfully. (*G–M*) Side-to-side anastomosis – antiperistaltic. (*K–M*) Antiperistaltic side-to-side anastomosis demonstrates 2 limbs of bowel adjacent to one another, often with sharply demarcated colonic and small bowel mucosa, which corresponds to the staple line. The stapled-off ends of the small and large bowel are encountered directly, whereas the proximal intestine is located behind the tip of the colonoscope. (*J*) This is evident on the fluoroscopic image of ileal intubation during colonoscopy of an antiperistaltic side-to-side anastomosis. (*L, M*)

long-term outcomes in postoperative CD patients.[26] The authors have found that the type of anastomosis has a significant impact on the long-term quality of life of patients, irrespective of recurrence of CD inflammation, with end-to-end anastomoses functioning better than side-to-side anastomoses (antiperistaltic orientation). In addition, the different types of anastomoses need to be accurately interpreted when assessing postoperative CD patients endoscopically. The underappreciation of different anastomotic configurations is apparent when considering that one of the major endoscopic reporting programs, ProVation (Minneapolis, Minnesota), offers only 1 diagram (**Fig. 2**P) for describing endoscopic findings in postoperative CD patients (although there are text dropdown menus to accurately describe anastomotic type and also a separate drop down menu to annotate the Rutgeerts ileal recurrence score). For gastroenterologists to take full advantage of endoscopic assessment of the surgery site, comprehensive understanding and command of the endoscopic appearance of the surgical anatomy after reconstruction are required. The 4 most common types of surgical reconstruction and endoscopic features are outlined and guidance provided on their clinical strengths and limitations from the perspective of the endoscopist.

End-to-End Ileocolonic Anastomosis

An end-to-end ileocolonic anastomosis is created when the intestine is reconstructed as an intact tube. This anastomosis is most commonly achieved with a hand-sewn approach, as shown in **Fig. 2**A–D. Stapling devices for an end-to-end connection are more commonly used in the anastomosis of an ileal J-pouch to the rectal cuff (double-stapled ileal pouch anal anastomosis) in patients with ulcerative colitis but are less commonly used in small bowel anastomosis. End-to-end anastomosis is technically more challenging due to the different luminal calibers between the small and large intestines or prestenotic segments of bowel, which are dilated in comparison to decompressed downstream segments. End-to-end anastomosis take significantly longer intraoperative time periods to achieve compared with a stapled side-to-side anastomosis, and this was demonstrated in a randomized head-to-head comparison trial between these 2 types of anastomoses.[27] Despite the technical challenges and the longer intraoperative time required, there was no difference in rates of complications between these 2 types of anastomoses. Creating an anastomosis often requires spatulation of the smaller caliber intestinal segment to achieve tissue apposition. The advantage of the end-to-end configuration is a restoration of the native intestinal physiology, which allows for optimal transmission of peristaltic contractions, which in turn does not interrupt the flow of bowel contents because the intestines contract in a monodirectional way. The intact tube reconstruction of an end-to-end anastomosis also works optimally to prevent stasis of enteric contents and bacterial overgrowth, both of which may further compromise clinical status in postoperative CD patients.

◀───

Stenosis at the antiperistaltic side to side most commonly occurs at the inlet and is best appreciated on a retroflex view. (*N*, *O*) Side-to-side anastomosis – isoperistaltic. In contrast to the antiperistaltic side-to-side anastomosis, the isoperistaltic side-to-side anastomosis has two lumens clearly visible, with proximal bowel visualized directly ahead during colonoscopy. (*P*) Representative diagram of an ileocolonic anastomosis on and endoscopic reporting system. This software does not offer specific diagrams for different ileocolonic anastomoses but does offer text to describe the different types of commonly encountered reconstructions. The numbers on the image correspond to endoscopic images of that bowel segment that have been selected for inclusion on the colonoscopy report.

New investigation from the authors' Inflammatory Bowel Disease Center at UPMC has suggested that the reconstruction of the intestine in a physiologic fashion with the end-to-end anastomosis results in significantly improved quality of life, less health care utilization (emergency room visits, hospitalizations, abdominal pelvic CT scans), and reduced health care charge expenditures in CD patients compared with individuals who have undergone a side-to-side, antiperistaltic anastomosis over the 2-year postoperative time period.[26] These prospective observational data in 128 patients from a single center did not demonstrate differences in postoperative recurrence of CD, complications associated with the surgery or differential treatment requirements with immunomodulatory, and/or biologic agents in the preoperative and postoperative time periods. These data suggest that the restoration of physiologic function translates into overall improved clinical status in CD patients, and, as a result of this comparative effectiveness study, the end-to-end anastomosis has emerged as the dominant procedure for CD reconstruction in the authors' institution.

Endoscopic assessment of the end-to-end anastomosis is readily achieved, because the anatomy is an intact tube, and this may be the easiest anastomosis to allow for deep intubation of the small bowel during colonoscopy. Endoscopic features of the anastomosis may include visible sutures (ie, silk ties that do not degrade) as well as the identification of the 2 different types of mucosa of the small bowel and colon that are found in a direct continuous fashion adjacent to each other. **Fig. 2**A–D displays a typical endoscopic appearance of an end-to-end anastomosis.

CD recurrence typically occurs at the proximal aspect of the end-to-end ileocolonic anastomosis or in the neoterminal ileum just above the anastomosis. Rutgeerts scoring of the end-to-end anastomosis frequently describes deeper regions of the proximal small intestine in addition to the area immediately proximal to the suture line. The hand-sewn end-to-end anastomosis is not readily apparent on radiographic studies, because the silk ties are not radio-opaque, unlike the metal staples routinely used in side-to-side anastomosis. Surgeons can help to mark anastomoses by placing metal clips in the mesentery adjacent to the anastomosis in a regimented fashion, which are apparent on routine radiographic studies.

Anastomotic strictures can form at the end-to-end anastomosis, and these typically occur in the area just proximal to the suture line, as seen in **Fig. 2**D. Early strictures, occurring within the first year after surgery, may be related to postoperative healing, forming a weblike configuration. If an anastomotic stricture is encountered (whether related to recurrent CD or to hypertrophied tissue/scar at the anastomosis), the option of endoscopic balloon dilatation of the stricture should be considered. Through the scope (TTS) balloons can be readily deployed under direct endoscopic vision across the anastomotic stricture. The end-to-end configuration allows for a relatively easy balloon dilatation because the anastomosis is encountered in direct position en face with no torque on the scope, as shown in **Fig. 2**A–D. Details regarding candidacy for TTS balloon dilatation are discussed later. In situations where TTS balloon dilatation is not favored, endoscopic visualization across the stricture or passage of a biopsy forceps across the strictured anastomosis into the neoterminal ileum can be considered. Multiple blind biopsies across the strictured anastomosis, however, are not highly recommended due to the potential for creating a perforation.

End-to-Side Ileocolonic Anastomosis

The end-to-side ileocolonic anastomosis can be achieved with either a hand-sewn or stapled approach (using a circular stapler). Historically, a hand-sewn end-to-side anastomosis was one of the more commonly performed procedures, because this would routinely allow for 2 different calibers of bowel to be reconstructed together and achieve continuity. Usually, the end-to-side anastomosis is created between the neoterminal ileum and the ascending colon as demonstrated in **Fig. 2**E. Surgical procedures prior to the 1980s would often favor a right hemicolectomy with an end-to-side ileocolonic anastomosis between the neoterminal ileum and the transverse colon at the hepatic flexure. Surgical intervention in the 1960s often emphasized an end-to-side anastomosis created in the midtransverse colon with the ascending colon left in place but excluded from the fecal stream. Thus, the vintage of the surgical procedure may provide important information regarding postoperative anatomy and the potential location of the end-to-side anastomosis. This is particularly challenging to identify endoscopically when the anastomosis lies distal to the most proximal segments of the remaining colon. The endoscopic appearance of the classic end-to-side ileocolonic anastomosis, which is constructed in proximity to the closed-off colonic segment, demonstrates a connection to the small bowel in a side wall distal to this base, as seen in **Fig. 2**E. The stapled end-to-side ileocolonic anastomosis frequently has a relatively small opening into the intestine, which may be related to the small opening of the circular stapling device used to create this connection into the side wall of the colon. The stapled end-to-side anastomosis can undergo balloon dilation, because this is often a web stricture immediately at the anastomotic site, as shown in **Fig. 2**F.

Given the limitations of the opening in the side wall and/or the more narrow opening of a stapled end-to-side anastomosis, deep endosopic cannulation of the proximal small intestine may be more difficult with this anastomotic configuration.

Side-to-Side Ileocolonic Anastomosis

At present, perhaps the most common anastomosis after ileocolonic resection is the stapled, antiperistaltic side-to-side anastomosis (**Fig. 2**G). Stapled anastomoses typically use a linear stapling device, which is designed to deploy 2 rows of titanium staples, which are then separated with a cutting blade. The common channel is then closed with a perpendicular staple line, which creates a right angle closure of the blind end of the anastomosis. Although no precise data are available regarding the specific rates of anastomosis types used at the present time, the recently published PREVENT trial, which was a multicenter, multinational trial assessing CD recurrence with and without biologic therapy, provides some insight.[22] Approximately half of the patients recruited to this trial had side-to-side anastomoses created at the discretion of their treating surgeons. The reasons underlying the recent dominance of the side-to-side anastomosis stem from the use of this technique in laparoscopic surgery where the anastomosis is being created intracorporally, which mandates that surgical stapling devices be used to create the reconstruction. Many laparascopic surgical procedures for CD, however, favor a laparoscopic dissection with the creation of a working incision, which allows bowel to be exteriorized and the anastomosis to be created extracorporally with either hand-sewn end-to-end or stapled side-to-side reconstruction.

The side-to-side anastomosis was originally developed by Soviet trauma surgeons in the 1950s due to the speed of this reconstructive approach, which is an essential tenet in trauma surgery. This type of anastomosis is the fastest of all reconstructions in the operating room and is often favored by surgeons for its speed and simplicity. The side-to-side anastomosis does not require a complex solution for 2 bowel lumens, which are not precisely the same caliber. The 2 segments of intestine are arranged next to one another and the stapling device is fired in a linear orientation. The anastomosis is closed with a perpendicular staple line, either across both limbs (antiperistaltic side-to-side anastomosis, as demonstrated in **Fig. 2**G) or over each limb individually (isoperistaltic side-to-side anastomosis, as in **Fig. 2**N). In the study by

McLeod and colleagues,[27] the stapled side-to-side anastomosis was significantly faster to build in the operating room, and the end-to-end anastomosis was essentially 3 times slower. In the Inflammatory Bowel Disease Center at UPMC, surgeons using a side-to-side anastomosis have an average operative time, which is 60 minutes faster than the end-to-end anastomosis.

Because of the nature of the bowel connection, the antiperistaltic side-to-side anastomosis forms a blind pouch where bowel contents pool. Movement of enteric contents is propelled by the movement of upstream material into the side-to-side anastomosis, which then pushes content downstream. Fecalization and distention are 2 potential adverse events, which can occur in the larger side-to-side anastomoses. In an attempt to further refine the antiperistaltic anastomotic configuration, surgeons have attempted to taper the blunt ends of this anastomosis using additional angled staple lines. This modification of the antiperistaltic side-to-side anastomosis is known as the functional end-to-end anastomosis.

Endoscopic assessment of the antiperistaltic side-to-side anastomosis or the functional end-to-end anastomosis demonstrates an unusual configuration where the endoscopist arrives at a bowel segment where there are essentially 2 bowel lumens next to one another (**Fig. 2H–M**). The 2 lumens are separated by a staple line, which often resembles the endoscopic configuration of a J-pouch, ileoanal reconstruction endoscopically with an owl's eye appearance. The endoscopist who enters an antiperistaltic side-to-side anastomosis needs to recognize this configuration to find the afferent intestine, which enters the anastomosis behind the area of visualization during colonoscopy. The endoscopist must retroflex the tip of the colonoscope to see the proximal small bowel, which enters the anastomosis (**Fig. 2J**). This is most challenging in the functional end-to-end anastomosis, which is typically constructed with contoured staple lines, which attempt to create less severe right angles at the anastomotic site. The side-to-side anastomosis can also be recognized endoscopically, by the appearance of 2 distinct types of mucosa – where colonic mucosa abuts a villous small bowel mucosa in a sharp demarcation corresponding with the staple line.

Endoscopists who are not familiar with the side-to-side antiperistaltic configuration of the anastomosis may be confused by the stapled-off blind ends that are encountered when entering the saclike structure. This can be misinterpreted as a stricture at the anastomosis, when the true lumen is behind the view of the endoscope. Having the skill to retroflex the tip of the endoscope within the side-to-side anastomosis is essential to visualize the upstream bowel. More importantly, endoscopic recurrence in the antiperistaltic side-to-side anastomosis occurs predictably at the inlet of the small bowel entering the anastomosis. It is rare to detect endoscopic activity at the staple line between the small and large bowel segments that have been anastomosed.

The isoperistaltic side-to-side ileocolonic anastomosis attempts to preserve an antegrade motility pattern as contents are propelled forward in line with the anastomosis (**Fig. 2N, O**). Both of these side-to-side anastomoses disrupt the circular smooth muscle layers, which are needed for normal peristaltic activity, and there is a potential for an a-motile sac–like configuration to form at the site of the anastomosis. Stasis of bowel contents across isoperistaltic anastomoses occurs less frequently than in cases where there is an antiperistaltic anastomosis.

ENDOSCOPIC BALLOON DILATION AND STEROID INJECTION IN ANASTOMOTIC STRICTURES

Postoperatively, CD patients are at risk for developing strictures at the site of the surgical anastomosis, which may often have a shallow, weblike configuration. Once an anastomotic stricture has formed, the use of medical therapy is of limited value and these strictures are best managed endoscopically with TTS balloon dilatation. The goal of TTS endoscopically guided balloon dilatation of the anastomotic stricture is to relieve symptoms of obstruction and to replace or postpone the need for yet another surgical resection. Balloon dilation may also be accompanied by intralesional steroid injection, which may further delay or prevent the need for repeat dilatation or surgical resection or stricturoplasty. When considering the efficacy of TTS endoscopic balloon treatment in the management of CD, dilatation of anastomotic strictures has the highest rates of success, which approaches 97% for immediate technical success, which indicates successful passage of the scope past the stricture after dilatation.[28–30] When evaluating the effect of TTS balloon dilatation on clinical efficacy, which was defined as resolution of the obstructive symptoms, success rates were as high as 100%.[31,32] Therefore, use of a TTS balloon dilatation attempt is preferred over referral for surgery, whenever possible.

There are no set guidelines regarding technical aspects of TTS endoscopic balloon dilatation of anastomotic strictures in CD. A pragmatic approach reserves TTS balloon dilatation for benign fibrotic strictures (not inflammatory) that are short (<4 cm in length) and that are not associated with fistulous tracts, abscesses, or malignancy. These strictures often do not allow passage of the tip of the adult colonoscope (diameter of 12.8 mm).[33–35] There are no set guidelines regarding the size of balloon dilatation to be performed, duration of balloon insufflation, graded dilation, antegrade versus retrograde, wire-guided versus non–wire-guided, intralesional injection of steroid, and the use of fluoroscopy to assist with the procedure. At the Inflammatory Bowel Disease Center, the choice of balloon is often based on the size of the stricture, where initial balloon choice is smaller than the tip of the colonoscope (which was unable to traverse the anastomotic stricture). In general, there is repeat balloon expansion across the stricture for 30 to 120 seconds, depending on the stricture diameter and endoscopist, with inspection of the site for assessment of immediate technical success. Published series have recommended maximum balloon dilation between 18 mm and 25 mm diameter, with a typical balloon diameter of 20 mm insufflated to 3 to 6 atm.[33,36]

Use of steroid injection after successful balloon dilation of an anastomotic stricture is based on the rationale that this treatment reduces scarring at the disrupted esophageal stricture after dilation. Triamcinolone acetonide injectable suspension (40 mg/mL) is the most commonly used steroid and is administered via endoscopic sclerotherapy needle in 4 quadrants at the postdilatation of the anastomotic site using 0.5 mL to 1.0 mL per injection.[29] Brooker and colleagues[37] reported a success rate of single steroid injection in 50% after dilation (median follow-up of 16.4 months), which rose to 78.6% when additional dilation/injections were performed (median follow-up of 27.8 months). In contrast, Atreja and colleagues[38] failed to demonstrate a difference in outcomes of anastomotic strictures that were treated with intralesional steroids. The results on the use of triamcinolone after balloon dilatation have been mixed, with some but not all studies suggesting a reduced need for repeat dilations. Some investigators have also advised caution regarding the use of intralesional injection of steroids after balloon dilatation in CD patients who are receiving biologic therapy (anti–tumor necrosis factor or anti-integrin agents), due to concern regarding an increased risk of infection.

In conclusion, TTS balloon dilatation is a relatively safe procedure that has shown promising results in CD patients with obstruction due to anastomotic stricture. Endoscopic balloon dilatation can achieve both short-term and long-term symptomatic improvement. Selection of strictures that are shallow and weblike offer the best outcome. Ideally, TTS balloon dilatation is performed electively and not in the emergent setting. Patients should understand the risks of perforation with this procedure, which have ranged from 2% to 18%.[39] CD patients undergoing balloon dilatation of an anastomotic stricture should be appropriate candidates for rescue surgery if it is required.

SUMMARY

In summary, endoscopic assessment of the ileocecal surgical anastomosis in CD is an essential diagnostic procedure that carries important prognostic significance. Advances in surgical techniques have led to the development of 4 anastomotic reconstructions, which are commonly encountered in clinical practice – the end-to-end anastomosis, the end-to-side anastomosis, the antiperistaltic side-to-side anastomosis, and the isoperistaltic side-to-side anastomosis. At present, surgical societies do not recommend one anastomotic configuration over another, leaving this choice to the discretion of the treating surgeon. This is based on data suggesting equivalent rates of complications and endoscopic recurrence at the anastomotic site. Emerging data suggest, however, that long-term clinical outcomes may be superior in CD patients who undergo end-to-end anastomosis, where improved quality of life and decreased health care utilization and health care expenditures were identified compared with patients who underwent an antiperistaltic side-to-side anastomosis. Gastroenterologists need to be familiar with the endoscopic appearance of these different types of anastomoses, because misinterpretation of the anatomy may inadvertently lead to description of stenosis at a blind limb of bowel, which is an expected finding in the side-to-side configuration. In addition to the diagnostic importance of correctly assessing the anastomotic configuration, postoperative assessment of CD recurrence guides early medical intervention with immunomodulator and/or biologic agents. Emerging data have demonstrated that early use of these agents in the postoperative time period may improve long-term clinical outcomes in patients with aggressive recurrence of CD at the anastomotic site. Finally, endoscopy can therapeutically address stricture formation at the anastomotic site with balloon dilatation, which can alleviate obstructive symptoms and obviate repeat resection.

REFERENCES

1. Crohn B, Ginzburg L, Oppenheimer G. Regional ileitis: a pathologic and clinical entity. JAMA 1932;99(16):1323–9.
2. Rutgeerts P, Geboes K, Vantrappen G, et al. Predictability of the postoperative course of Crohn's disease. Gastroenterology 1990;99(4):956–63.
3. De Cruz P, Kamm MA, Hamilton AL, et al. The First Validated Post-Operative Endoscopic Crohns Disease Index: The POCER Index. Identification of Key Endoscopic Prognostic Factors. Gastroenterology. April 2016;150(4), Supplement 1, p. S–72.
4. Hanauer SB, Korelitz BI, Rutgeerts P, et al. Postoperative maintenance of Crohn's disease remission with 6-mercaptopurine, mesalamine, or placebo: a 2-year trial. Gastroenterology 2004;127(3):723–9.
5. D'Haens GR, Vermeire S, Van Assche G, et al. Therapy of metronidazole with azathioprine to prevent postoperative recurrence of Crohn's disease: a controlled randomized trial. Gastroenterology 2008;135(4):1123–9.
6. Herfarth H, Tjaden C, Lukas M, et al. Adverse events in clinical trials with azathioprine and mesalamine for prevention of postoperative recurrence of Crohn's disease. Gut 2006;55(10):1525–6.

7. Rutgeerts P, Hiele M, Geboes K, et al. Controlled trial of metronidazole treatment for prevention of Crohn's recurrence after ileal resection. Gastroenterology 1995; 108(6):1617–21.

8. Rutgeerts P, Van Assche G, Vermeire S, et al. Ornidazole for prophylaxis of post-operative Crohn's disease recurrence: a randomized, double-blind, placebo-controlled trial. Gastroenterology 2005;128(4):856–61.

9. Florent C, Cortot A, Quandale P, et al. Placebo-controlled clinical trial of mesalazine in the prevention of early endoscopic recurrences after resection for Crohn's disease. Groupe d'Etudes Therapeutiques des Affections Inflammatoires Digestives (GETAID). Eur J Gastroenterol Hepatol 1996;8(3):229–33.

10. Caprilli R, Andreoli A, Capurso L, et al. Oral mesalazine (5-aminosalicylic acid; Asacol) for the prevention of post-operative recurrence of Crohn's disease. Gruppo Italiano per lo Studio del Colon e del Retto (GISC). Aliment Pharmacol Ther 1994;8(1):35–43.

11. Caprilli R, Cottone M, Tonelli F, et al. Two mesalazine regimens in the prevention of the post-operative recurrence of Crohn's disease: a pragmatic, double-blind, randomized controlled trial. Aliment Pharmacol Ther 2003; 17(4):517–23.

12. Regueiro M, Schraut W, Baidoo L, et al. Infliximab prevents Crohn's disease recurrence after ileal resection. Gastroenterology 2009;136(2):441–50.e1 [quiz: 716].

13. Sorrentino D, Terrosu G, Avellini C, et al. Infliximab with low-dose methotrexate for prevention of postsurgical recurrence of ileocolonic Crohn's disease. Arch Intern Med 2007;167(16):1804–7.

14. Yoshida K, Fukunaga K, Ikeuchi H, et al. Scheduled infliximab monotherapy to prevent recurrence of Crohn's disease following ileocolic or ileal resection: a 3-year prospective randomized open trial. Inflamm Bowel Dis 2012;18(9):1617–23.

15. Armuzzi A, Felice C, Papa A, et al. Prevention of postoperative recurrence with azathioprine or infliximab in patients with Crohn's disease: an open-label pilot study. J Crohns Colitis 2013;7(12):e623–9.

16. Fernández-Blanco IMJ, Martinez B, Cara C, et al. Adalimumab in the prevention of postoperative recurrence of Crohn's disease. Gastroenterology 2010; 138(5 Suppl 1):S-692.

17. Papamichael K, Archavlis E, Lariou C, et al. Adalimumab for the prevention and/or treatment of post-operative recurrence of Crohn's disease: a prospective, two-year, single center, pilot study. J Crohns Colitis 2012;6(9):924–31.

18. Savarino E, Dulbecco P, Bodini G, et al. Prevention of postoperative recurrence of Crohn's disease by Adalimumab: a case series. Eur J Gastroenterol Hepatol 2012;24(4):468–70.

19. Aguas M, Bastida G, Cerrillo E, et al. Adalimumab in prevention of postoperative recurrence of Crohn's disease in high-risk patients. World J Gastroenterol 2012; 18(32):4391–8.

20. Savarino E, Bodini G, Dulbecco P, et al. Adalimumab is more effective than azathioprine and mesalamine at preventing postoperative recurrence of Crohn's disease: a randomized controlled trial. Am J Gastroenterol 2013;108(11): 1731–42.

21. De Cruz P, Kamm MA, Hamilton AL, et al. Crohn's disease management after intestinal resection: a randomised trial. Lancet 2015;385(9976):1406–17.

22. Regueiro M, Feagan BG, Zou B, et al. Infliximab Reduces Endoscopic, but Not Clinical, Recurrence of Crohn's Disease After Ileocolonic Resection. Gastroenterol 2016;150(7):1568–78.

23. Hashash JG, Regueiro M. A practical approach to preventing postoperative recurrence in Crohn's disease. Curr Gastroenterol Rep 2016;18(5):25.

24. Hashash JG, Regueiro M. The evolving management of postoperative Crohn's disease. Expert Rev Gastroenterol Hepatol 2012;6(5):637–48.

25. Strong S, Steele SR, Boutrous M, et al. Clinical practice guideline for the surgical management of Crohn's disease. Dis Colon Rectum 2015;58(11):1021–36.

26. Gajendran M, Watson AR, Bauer AJ, et al. End to end vs side to side anastomosis and post-operative Crohn's disease quality of life and healthcare utilization: A prospective comparative effectiveness study. Gastroenterology 2015;148(4 Suppl 1):S-177.

27. McLeod RS, Wolff BG, Ross S, et al. Investigators of the CAST trial. Recurrence of Crohn's disease after ileocolic resection is not affected by anastomotic type: results of a multicenter, randomized, controlled trial. Dis Colon Rectum 2009;52(5): 919–27.

28. Stienecker K, Gleichmann D, Neumayer U, et al. Long-term results of endoscopic balloon dilatation of lower gastrointestinal tract strictures in Crohn's disease: a prospective study. World J Gastroenterol 2009;15(21):2623–7.

29. Singh VV, Draganov P, Valentine J. Efficacy and safety of endoscopic balloon dilation of symptomatic upper and lower gastrointestinal Crohn's disease strictures. J Clin Gastroenterol 2005;39(4):284–90.

30. Thienpont C, D'Hoore A, Vermeire S, et al. Long-term outcome of endoscopic dilatation in patients with Crohn's disease is not affected by disease activity or medical therapy. Gut 2010;59(3):320–4.

31. Matsui T, Hatakeyama S, Ikeda K, et al. Long-term outcome of endoscopic balloon dilation in obstructive gastroduodenal Crohn's disease. Endoscopy 1997;29(7):640–5.

32. Ramboer C, Verhamme M, Dhondt E, et al. Endoscopic treatment of stenosis in recurrent Crohn's disease with balloon dilation combined with local corticosteroid injection. Gastrointest Endosc 1995;42(3):252–5.

33. Paine E, Shen B. Endoscopic therapy in inflammatory bowel diseases (with videos). Gastrointest Endosc 2013;78(6):819–35.

34. Chen M, Shen B. Endoscopic therapy in Crohn's disease: principle, preparation, and technique. Inflamm Bowel Dis 2015;21(9):2222–40.

35. Hommes DW, van Deventer SJ. Endoscopy in inflammatory bowel diseases. Gastroenterology 2004;126(6):1561–73.

36. Hassan C, Zullo A, De Francesco V, et al. Systematic review: endoscopic dilatation in Crohn's disease. Aliment Pharmacol Ther 2007;26(11–12):1457–64.

37. Brooker JC, Beckett CG, Saunders BP, et al. Long-acting steroid injection after endoscopic dilation of anastomotic Crohn's strictures may improve the outcome: a retrospective case series. Endoscopy 2003;35(4):333–7.

38. Atreja A, Aggarwal A, Dwivedi S, et al. Safety and efficacy of endoscopic dilation for primary and anastomotic Crohn's disease strictures. J Crohns Colitis 2014; 8(5):392–400.

39. Makkar R, Shen B. Colonoscopic perforation in inflammatory bowel disease. Gastroenterol Hepatol 2013;9(9):573–83.

The Gastroenterologist's Role in Management of Perianal Fistula

 CrossMark

Robin L. Dalal, MD[a], David A. Schwartz, MD[b],*

KEYWORDS

- Perianal • Crohn's disease • Fistula • Combination therapy

KEY POINTS

- Perianal Crohn's disease is common and carries significant morbidity for patients.
- Medical and surgical therapy for perianal fistula has improved greatly.
- Endoscopy plays a role as an adjunct to medical and surgical management of fistulizing perianal Crohn's disease.
- Currently, a multidisciplinary approach to complex perianal fistulas is believed to lead to the best outcomes.

INTRODUCTION

Perianal fistulas are common in the Crohn's disease population and can be disabling to patients. Knowledge of fistulizing Crohn's disease has grown immensely over the past 75 years and therapies have improved greatly. This article reviews fistulizing Crohn's disease and examines the current strategies of management including medications, endoscopy, and surgical care.

ANATOMY

Before embarking on a discussion of perianal fistulizing disease, it is important to understand the anatomy of the area. Perianal anatomy is complex and involves the pelvic floor musculature and the gastrointestinal tract. As seen in **Fig. 1**, the anal canal is composed of epithelial lining, subepithelium, supporting tissues with intertwining neuronal networks, and specialized musculature including the pelvic floor and anal sphincter complex.[1] Within the lumen, the upper anal canal is composed of the transitional and columnar epithelium of the rectum. This changes to the squamous anal

[a] Division of Gastroenterology, Vanderbilt University Medical Center, 1600 The Vanderbilt Clinic, Nashville, TN 37232-5280, USA; [b] Division of Gastroenterology, Vanderbilt University Medical Center, Suite 220, 1211 21st Avenue, Nashville, TN 37232, USA
* Corresponding author.
E-mail address: David.a.schwartz@vanderbilt.edu

Gastrointest Endoscopy Clin N Am 26 (2016) 693–705
http://dx.doi.org/10.1016/j.giec.2016.06.008
1052-5157/16/© 2016 Elsevier Inc. All rights reserved.

giendo.theclinics.com

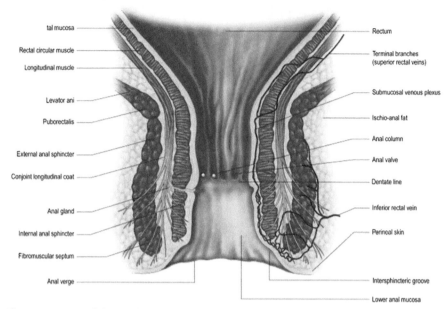

Fig. 1. Anatomy of the anal canal. (*From* Standring S. Lower intestine. In: Standring S, editor. Gray's anatomy, vol. 41. Philadelphia: Elsevier; 2016. p. 1136–59; with permission.)

epithelium at the dentate line. At the dentate line, there are anal columns and crypts. The bases of crypts may contain anal glands that then may penetrate the supporting tissues including the intersphincteric space. The anal sphincter complex is composed of the internal anal sphincter and the external anal sphincter. The internal anal sphincter is the thickened terminal extension of the circular muscle of the rectum and the external anal sphincter is a tube of striated muscle extending from the puborectalis muscle. **Fig. 2** shows the interplay of the sphincter complex and the rest of the pelvic floor.

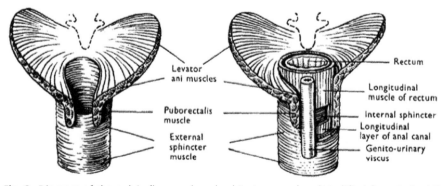

Fig. 2. Diagram of the pelvic floor and anal sphincter complex. (*Modified from* Parks AG, Gordon PH, Hardcastle JD. A classification of fistula-in-ano. Br J Surg 1976;63(1):1–12; with permission.)

EPIDEMIOLOGY

The first record of a granulomatous fistula was made by Gabriel[2] in 1921 during a series of histologic investigations of 75 patients with rectal fistulae. In setting out to examine fistulae related to tuberculosis, he discovered that there were some fistulae with granulomas without evidence of tubercle bacilli. In 1932, Crohn's and Ginzburg's[3] original paper describing regional ileitis did not mention perianal fistulas. Bissell[4] in 1934 and Penner and Crohn's[5] in 1938 were the first to describe cases of patients with the clinical entity of Crohn's disease and concomitant perianal fistulae. Morson and Lockhart-Mummery[6] then described the histologic noncaseating giant-cell lesions in perianal fistulae to be similar to those seen in luminal Crohn's disease in 1959. After this, further case series in the 1960s and 1970s firmly established that perianal fistulae could be a manifestation of Crohn's disease.[7,8]

Since the original descriptions of perianal Crohn's disease, multiple population-based and referral-center-based studies have shown that perianal disease is common. In population-based studies from the United States, Canada, and Sweden, the rates of perianal fistulas in patients with Crohn's disease range from 21% to 28%.[9–12] Referral-center-based studies cite frequencies of perianal fistulas ranging from 22% to 40% in patients with Crohn's disease.[9,13–15] Perianal disease has been found to be more common in patients with distal luminal Crohn's disease, such as colonic or ileocolonic disease, versus isolated ileal disease.[10,11] The risk of developing a perianal fistula increases over time after diagnosis of Crohn's disease with a 21% cumulative risk after 10 years and a 26% cumulative risk after 20 years as seen in **Fig. 3.**[9] It is also important to note that perianal disease can be the only manifestation of Crohn's disease in about 5% of patients.[9]

This population of patients has also been found to have slightly different characteristics than other patients with Crohn's disease. Patients with perianal disease have more disabling Crohn's disease after 5 years of diagnosis, especially if they also require steroids and are younger than the age of 40 at diagnosis.[16] A recent cross-sectional analysis of 333 patients with Crohn's disease on infliximab found that patients with perianal fistulas were almost three times more likely to be African American or Hispanic than white.[17] Patients with perianal fistula are more likely to have extraintestinal manifestations of their inflammatory bowel disease, such as arthritis, oral ulcerations, or skin manifestations.[13] They are more likely to develop penetrating or

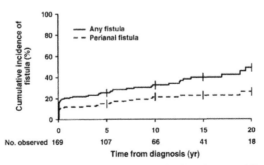

Fig. 3. Cumulative incidence of overall fistulas (*solid line*) and perianal fistulas (*dashed line*) among 176 Olmsted County, Minnesota residents diagnosed with Crohn's disease from 1970 to 1993. (*Modified from* Schwartz DA, Loftus EV, Tremaine WJ, et al. The natural history of fistulizing Crohn's disease in Olmsted County, Minnesota. Gastroenterology 2002;122(4): 875–80.)

structuring complications including a five-fold increased risk of developing a luminal fistula and a two-fold increased risk of requiring surgery.[11,12,15] Finally, patients are 2.3 times more likely to be steroid resistant if they have perianal disease.[18]

PATHOGENESIS

The cause of perianal fistulas in Crohn's disease is not entirely clear; however, multiple theories exist. One of the oldest theories of fistula pathogenesis involves a mucosal defect, such as a persistent infection or ulceration that then penetrates through the wall of the anal canal.[19] After the track is established, it is then thought that the pressure of the fecal stream maintains this opening.[20] Although the initial mucosal defect from this theory is thought to initiate fistula formation, the mechanical forces of the fecal material is what has been thought to perpetuate the fistula itself.[20] Another theory proposes that infection in the anal glands themselves is a cause of fistula.[19] Anatomically, the glands have ducts that can penetrate the internal anal sphincter and promote spread of infection into the intersphincteric space, the external anal sphincter, or even to the skin. On a cellular level, it is thought that the epithelial-to-mesenchymal transition (EMT) plays a role in fistula formation.[21] EMT is a process whereby an epithelial cell loses its defining properties including certain cell contacts and polarity and takes on mesenchymal cell properties including motility and migration. EMT occurs physiologically during organ development and wound healing and pathologically in tumor growth and fibrosis.[21] In Crohn's disease fistula tissue studies, cytokine profiles (increased transforming growth factor-β, interleukin-13) and increased matrix remodeling enzyme concentration support the idea that EMT plays a role.[21]

CLASSIFICATION

Multiple classification systems have been used to define and describe the extent of a patient's perianal disease. It is important to know classification and apply this to patients because treatment algorithms depend on correct classification. It also allows for a common language between gastroenterologists and surgeons in describing fistula anatomy. The simplest and oldest classification includes defining the fistula as high or low based on the dentate line.[22] A fistula that enters the rectum above the dentate line is considered a high fistula, whereas one that opens below the dentate line is a low fistula. Through further characterization of the anal canal and fistulas, additional more complex classification systems were developed. Two classifications are currently widely used, the Parks classification and the American Gastroenterological Association proposed classification system. The Parks classification was developed by Parks and colleagues[23] in 1976 and uses the external anal sphincter as the main point of reference for five main groups of fistulae. Fistulas are sorted into intersphincteric, transsphincteric, suprasphincteric, extrasphincteric, and superficial. Intersphincteric fistulas do not involve the external anal sphincter and also fit with the previously described low fistula. Transsphincteric fistulas pass through the external anal sphincter. Suprasphincteric fistulas pass over the external anal sphincter and through the pelvic floor muscles (puborectalis, levator ani). Finally, extrasphincteric fistulas are outside the external sphincter complex altogether and pass through the rectal wall, pelvic floor muscles, and ischiorectal fossa.[23] Superficial fistulas do not involve either the internal or external sphincter. In the 2003 American Gastroenterological Association technical review of perianal fistulas, an additional classification was proposed combining physical examination and endoscopic evaluation to categorize fistulas as simple or complex.[24] Here, a simple fistula would be one that occurs low in the anal canal with a single external opening and no evidence of perianal abscess, rectovaginal fistula, or anorectal stricture. A complex fistula has a high origin above the dentate line; involves a significant portion of the external anal sphincter; and may have multiple external openings, pain, evidence of abscess, rectovagnial fistula, and stricture; and may have active rectal luminal disease on endoscopy.[24]

EVOLUTION OF THE ROLE OF THE GASTROENTEROLOGIST

Throughout the history of perianal Crohn's disease, the gastroenterologist's role has evolved from bystander to complex caregiver. In the 1970s, the management of perianal fistulas involved either observation or surgery.[8,20] Fistulas were observed if asymptomatic. If treated, fistulas were either surgically laid-open or drained. Rectal excision was also performed in certain cases.[8] In the 1980s, it was recognized that perianal lesions may heal if luminal Crohn's disease was successfully treated and that antibiotics may be beneficial; however, direct surgical management was still the mainstay of treatment, especially if there was evidence of an abscess. During this time, diversion of the fecal stream with either an elemental diet or a loop ileostomy was controversial but becoming popular.[25] By the 1990s, surgical therapy had advanced to include drainage, fistulotomy, fistulectomy, seton placement, mucosal flaps, fecal diversion, and proctectomy.[26] In a review of 224 patients with anorectal complications of Crohn's disease from 1984 to 1999, a total of 200 patients underwent surgical procedures for management of their disease and patients with active rectal disease were noted to have a higher rate of proctectomy.[27] With the advent of these more advanced surgical procedures, and knowledge of disease, medications, and detailed noninvasive tools, the gastroenterologist's role has changed. Currently, the gastroenterologist participates in diagnosis, investigation, and classification of disease through endoscopic assessment of luminal disease, endoscopic ultrasound (EUS) assessment of the perianal area, and coordination with radiologists for other imaging modalities. The gastroenterologist also directly manages medical therapy including biologic therapy and antibiotics. Finally, the gastroenterologist participates in coordination of care with surgical colleagues.

DIAGNOSIS AND INVESTIGATION OF PERIANAL DISEASE

Accurate diagnosis of the perianal process allows the gastroenterologist to classify fistulas appropriately and apply evidence-based care to patients. Diagnosis should involve a detailed examination, imaging, clinical assessment, and assessment of rectal inflammation.

The gold standard for diagnosis of perianal fistula has been the examination under anesthesia (EUA). Performed by a surgeon, the examination involves a digital rectal examination in combination with probing of the perianal area to define fistula tracts. For many years, management decisions regarding perianal Crohn's disease relied solely on the EUA. However, correct identification of all present abnormalities during EUA is difficult. A study by Van Beers and colleagues[28] in 1994 showed that accuracy of a digital rectal examination to define fistulas was only around 62%. Radiologic advances have allowed further investigation into fistulous networks and identification of more complex fistulas or perianal abscesses. Therefore, imaging is now an integral part of the diagnosis of fistulizing disease. Imaging modalities used in perianal Crohn's disease include fistulography, computed tomography, MRI, and EUS. Fistulography was the first imaging modality used. This involves injecting a small amount of radiopaque contrast into the fistula tract via a catheter that is inserted into the external fistula opening. This modality, however, has not been found to be extremely helpful, with only 16% to 50% accuracy when compared with operative findings; therefore its use has fallen out of favor.[29] Computed tomography has also proven to be unreliable for baseline evaluation of fistulous networks with an accuracy of 24% to 60% because of poor spatial resolution in the pelvis and inflammation that may cloud the image.[30] Computed tomography is, however, useful to identify secondary complications of perianal Crohn's disease, such as abscesses.

MRI and EUS have been shown to accurately diagnose fistulas and therefore have become the imaging modalities of choice in fistulizing Crohn's disease. Both modalities have similar accuracies ranging from 75% to 100% in multiple studies.[31–34] In a study of 34 patients with perianal fistulas comparing EUS, MRI, and EUA, the accuracy of all three modalities included EUS at 91%, MRI at 87%, and EUA at 91%.[35] For the patient, any of these imaging modalities is sufficient and the decision on which to use depends on the local expertise of the gastroenterologist. If high-quality EUS is available, it can be performed at the time of standard endoscopic evaluation of luminal disease activity. Using an imaging modality, such as MRI or EUS, has been shown to improve outcomes for patients. Combining two modalities of diagnosis (EUS, EUA, or MRI) led to an accuracy of 100%.[35] In a randomized study, patients who underwent EUA with EUS guidance had improved healing of disease versus patients who had EUA alone.[36] In addition to their usefulness in diagnosis, EUS and MRI are also integral to surveillance of fistulizing disease. A single-center experience reported in 2012 noted that follow-up EUS influenced patient management in 86% of its patients with perianal Crohn's disease.[37]

Objective scores of clinical activity can be gathered using the Perianal Disease Activity Index, which uses a Likert scale to rate specific metrics of quality of life and perianal disease severity.[38] Luminal activity should be assessed with standard endoscopy, such as flexible sigmoidoscopy. This is important because active inflammation may affect any available surgical options for treatment.[39]

Our suggestion for the gastroenterologist in investigation of patients with symptoms of fistulizing Crohn's disease is as follows: (1) perform a detailed history and physical examination, (2) perform endoscopy to assess disease activity, (3) perform either EUS or MRI as an imaging study to map out the fistulous process, and (4) refer for EUA for complete diagnosis and possible treatments.

MEDICAL MANAGEMENT THROUGH THE YEARS

The evolution of medical management of perianal Crohn's disease mirrors the progression of medical management of luminal disease. The first medications for fistulizing Crohn's disease were antibiotics, and their use has been propagated by multiple uncontrolled studies showing their benefit. Metronidazole was first reported as a treatment in 1977 in a small study where two patients had perianal Crohn's disease and improved dramatically after 6 months of metronidazole.[40] Bernstein and coworkers[41] in 1980 specifically studied 21 patients with perianal Crohn's disease and noted improved symptoms in all patients and complete healing in more than 50% of patients.

There are few controlled trials of antibiotics in perianal Crohn's disease; however, they have solidified the use of antibiotics in most patients with perianal fistulizing. The first controlled trial was performed in 2009. In this study, patients who were on concomitant therapy with either an immunomodulator or steroids were given placebo, ciprofloxacin, or metronidazole for 10 weeks. Closure of all open actively draining fistulas occurred in 30% of patients receiving either ciprofloxacin or metronidazole versus 12.5% in patients receiving placebo. Improvement in fistula drainage occurred in 54% of patients receiving either antibiotic versus 12.5% in patients receiving placebo.[42] However, this study was underpowered to detect a statistical difference in treatment arms because of lack of enrollment. A more recent randomized controlled trial involving combination antibiotics and anti–tumor necrosis factor (TNF) therapy was published in 2014. In this study, 76 patients with Crohn's disease with active perianal fistulas who were on maintenance adalimumab (40 mg every other week) were given ciprofloxacin, 500 mg twice daily, or placebo twice daily for 12 weeks. The ciprofloxacin/adalimumab group had statistically significant responses in clinical response (>50% fistula closure, 71% combination group and 47% placebo group) and remission (complete fistula closure, 65% combination group and 33% placebo group) during the study period. At Week 24 follow-up, however, after ciprofloxacin was removed, there were no differences in clinical response.[43]

Immunomodulator medications were the next medications used in perianal Crohn's disease. No prospective trials exist in evaluating azathioprine (AZA) or 6-mercaptopurine (6-MP) with fistula closure as a primary end point; however, their use is based on a meta-analysis of five controlled trials in which fistula closure was a secondary end point and uncontrolled case series in adults and children. The pooled odds ratio for fistula closure was 4.44.[44] When AZA or 6-MP have been combined with antibiotics in case series, patients have had even higher likelihood of achieving fistula closure or decreased drainage.[45] Methotrexate was shown to promote fistula closure or decreased drainage in a 2003 study of 33 patients who had failed or were intolerant of AZA or 6-MP.[46]

Multiple uncontrolled case series have shown that tacrolimus may be beneficial for fistula treatment. For example, tacrolimus combined with AZA or 6-MP in a small study of 11 patients from 1996 to 1998 resulted in clinical improvement in all patients and complete fistula closure in 64%.[47] The only randomized controlled study for tacrolimus was performed in 2003 in 48 patients with perianal or enterocutneous fistulas where 43% of tacrolimus-treated patients had fistula improvement compared with 8% of placebo-treated patients but not remission.[48] Topical tacrolimus has not been shown to improve fistulas despite the attractive idea that could save a patient from the adverse events of systemic tacrolimus.[49] Cyclosporine, which is similar in mechanism of action to tacrolimus, has also been used in fistulizing Crohn's disease in many uncontrolled case series where it overall has had an initial response rate of 83% but also had a high relapse rate when medication was discontinued.[24]

Similar to luminal Crohn's disease, the advent of biologic therapy significantly changed the management of perianal Crohn's disease. The anti-TNF-α antibody medications infliximab, adalimumab, and certolizumab have been studied in prospective controlled trials for perianal Crohn's disease. For infliximab, the first drug in this class, there have been two trials. The first trial, published in 1999 by Present and colleagues,[50] showed significant response of induction therapy with infliximab. Ninety-four patients were given placebo; 5 mg/kg infliximab at Weeks 0, 2, and 6; or 10 mg/kg infliximab at Weeks 0, 2, and 6. A total of 68% of patients in the 5 mg/kg group and 56% of patients in the 10 mg/kg group achieved the primary end point of greater than 50% reduction in number of draining fistulas compared with 26% of the placebo patients. The ACCENT II trial evaluated infliximab maintenance therapy for fistulizing Crohn's disease in 306 patients and showed that patients who received infliximab every 8 weeks for 1 year were more likely to have closure of fistulas than placebo (36%–19%).[51] A secondary analysis of this trial showed that infliximab maintenance also reduced hospitalizations, length of stay, and number of surgical procedures.[52]

Adalimumab is the second anti-TNF approved for Crohn's disease and has also shown efficacy in fistula healing. In the CHARM trial by Colombel and colleagues,[53] patients with fistulas achieved complete closure when treated with adalimumab versus placebo at Weeks 26 and 56 (30% adalimumab vs 13% placebo at Week 26, and 33% adalimumab vs 13% placebo at Week 56). In addition, for the patients who had complete fistula closure at Week 26, a total of 100% of them maintained closure at 56 weeks. At the end of the CHARM study period, the subgroup of patients with draining baseline fistulas were then followed for an additional year in an open-label extension study (ADHERE). In this study, complete fistula healing was sustained for the additional year (total 2 years of adalimumab) in 90% of patients.[54]

Certolizumab is the final biologic anti-TNF therapy with current evidence showing efficacy in perianal fistula healing. A total of 108 patients with draining fistulas from the PreCise 2 trial received open-label induction with certolizumab and were assessed at 6 months. At 6 months, 36% of the patients receiving certolizumab had fistula closure compared with 17% of placebo.[55]

The newest biologic medication, vedolizumab, was approved for Crohn's disease in 2014 and there currently are limited data in regards to perianal Crohn's disease. In a small cohort of patients within the phase III clinical trial of induction and maintenance of vedolizumab, fistula closure was achieved at Week 52 in 41.2% of patients who were maintained on vedoliuzmab every 8 weeks compared with 11.1% of patients who received placebo.[56]

COMBINING THERAPIES

Our current management of complex perianal Crohn's disease combines medical and surgical therapy. The first iterations of combined therapy in perianal Crohn's disease occurred with combining surgical therapy with antibiotics to decrease septic complications.[25,57] As medical therapy advanced, the logical addition of immunosuppressive medications, such as AZA and 6-MP (or tacrolimus and cyclosporine in selected patients), occurred with ongoing surgical treatments. The concept of dedicated combination therapy in complex fistulas came about in the era of biologic therapy after infliximab was shown in placebo-controlled trials to be effective in fistula healing. Initially, there was some controversy between gastroenterologists and surgeons as to the appropriate first-line therapy (infliximab vs seton placement); however, through the years it has become accepted that biologic therapy with combined surgical treatment leads to the best outcomes in patients. Multiple small retrospective studies support this practice. For example, combining EUA with possible seton placement and infliximab therapy was shown to lead to a better initial response, lower recurrence rate, and longer time to recurrence in 32 patients at a single center in Pittsburgh.[58] In Canada, it was also shown that selective seton placement combined with infliximab in 29 patients led to complete healing in 67% of patients.[59]

CURRENT MANAGEMENT

The current management of fistulizing perianal Crohn's disease depends on the type of fistula and the assessment of rectal inflammation.[30,38,39,59–61] The gastroenterologist should proceed with diagnostic evaluation as outlined previously and with that information decide on appropriate therapeutic options. A suggested algorithm is shown in **Fig. 4**. The first division of patients occurs when defining a patient with a simple versus a complex fistula.

Simple fistulas can be managed first with medical therapy, but must further be stratified according to active proctitis. In the patient with a simple fistula and no proctitis, antibiotics and immunomodulator therapy should be instituted. If this fails, then surgical therapy with simple fistulotomy should be tried. If rectal inflammation is present,

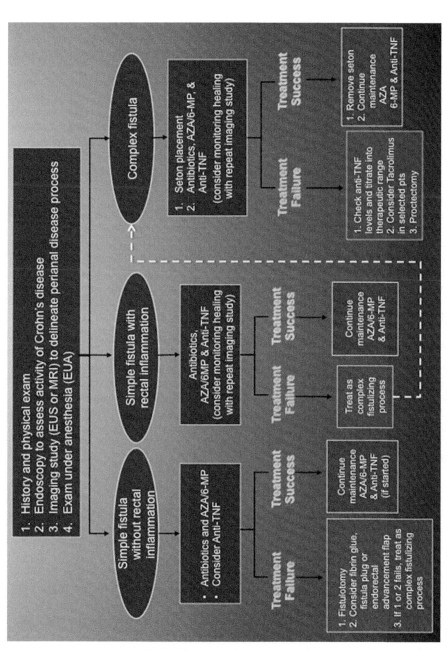

Fig. 4. Algorithm for diagnosis and management of perianal fistulizing Crohn's disease.

then anti-TNF therapy should be added as first-line to reduce inflammation and promote fistula healing.[38,39]

Complex fistulas require more intense treatment from the start to improve quality of life and reduce the chance for protectomy. Patients should have combined medical and surgical treatment at the onset with seton placement, antibiotic, and anti-TNF therapy. The goal of a noncutting seton is to allow the medical therapy to be more effective by preventing premature closure of the cutaneous side of the fistula tract, which could lead to abscess and sepsis.[39]

Refractory fistulas unfortunately occur in some patients and the available options at this point are surgical therapies including collagen plugs, fibrin glue, fecal diversion, flap repair, stem cell therapy, and proctocolectomy. Plug therapy involves inserting a collagen plug into the intestinal opening of the fistula. Fibrin glue insertion involves insertion of glue (composed of a combination of factors promoting activation of thrombin for clot formation) directly into the fistula tract during EUA. It has been shown to be effective in controlled trials; for example, in a study of fibrin glue in 34 patients not on anti-TNF therapy, 38% achieved remission versus 16% in the placebo group.[62] Surgical fecal diversion may assist in healing; however, recurrence is common after takedown. Mucosal advancement flap involves mobilization of the rectal mucosal flap to close the internal fistula opening. There have been reported success rate around 64%; however, half of patients need reintervention.[38] Stem-cell therapy involves local administration of stem cells into fistulous tracts. This therapy has been shown in small placebo-controlled trials to be safe and promising with healing in up to 85% of patients; larger trials are underway.[63,64] Finally, protectomy is the most definitive treatment of perianal Crohn's disease and is reserved for patients who fail all other medical and surgical options.

SUMMARY

Perianal Crohn's disease can be debilitating for patients with Crohn's disease and may require multidisciplinary therapy. The gastroenterologist serves as the investigator with baseline endoscopy and possible EUS. He or she also serves as the coordinator of care and after thorough evaluation, should work with surgeons and radiologists to allow for the best chance of healing for patients.

REFERENCES

1. Birch R. Anal canal. In: Standring S, editor. Gray's anatomy, vol. 41. Elsevier; 2016. p. 1136–59.
2. Gabriel WB. Results of an experimental and histological investigation into seventy-five cases of rectal fistulae. Proc R Soc Med 1921;14:156–61.
3. Crohn B, Ginzburg LOG. Regional ileitis; a pathologic and clinical entity. J Am Med Assoc 1932;99(16):1323–9.
4. Bissell AD. Localized chronic ulcerative ileitis. Ann Surg 1934;99(6):957–66. Available at: http://www.pubmedcentral.nih.gov/articlerender.fcgi?artid=1390067&tool=pmcentrez&rendertype=abstract.
5. Penner A, Crohn BB. Perianal fistulae as a complication of regional ileitis. Ann Surg 1938;108(5):867–73.
6. Morson BC, Lockhart-Mummery H. Anal lesions in Crohn's disease. Lancet 1959; 2:1122–3.
7. Gray BK, Lockhart-mummery HE, Morson BC. Crohn's disease of the anal region. Gut 1965;6(6):515–24.

8. Marks C, Ritchie J, Lockhart-Mummery H. Anal fistulas in Crohn's disease. Br J Surg 1976;63(1):1–12.

9. Schwartz DA, Loftus EV, Tremaine WJ, et al. The natural history of fistulizing Crohn's disease in Olmsted County, Minnesota. Gastroenterology 2002;122(4): 875–80.

10. Hellers G, Bergstrand O, Ewerth S, et al. Occurrence and outcome after primary treatment of anal fistulae in Crohn's disease. Gut 1980;21(6):525–7.

11. Tang LY, Rawsthorne P, Bernstein CN. Are perineal and luminal fistulas associated in Crohn's disease? A population-based study. Clin Gastroenterol Hepatol 2006;4(9):1130–4.

12. Thia KT, Sandborn WJ, Harmsen WS, et al. Risk factors associated with progression to intestinal complications of Crohn's disease in a population-based cohort. Gastroenterology 2010;139(4):1147–55.

13. Rankin GB, Watts HD, Melnyk CS, et al. National cooperative Crohn's disease study: extraintestinal manifestations and perianal complications. Gastroenterology 1979;77(4 Pt 2):914–20.

14. Williams DR, Coller JA, Corman ML, et al. Anal complications in Crohn's disease. Dis Colon Rectum 1981;24(1):22–4.

15. Lapidus A, Bernell O, Hellers G, et al. Clinical course of colorectal Crohn's disease: a 35-year follow-up study of 507 patients. Gastroenterology 1998;114(6):1151–60.

16. Beaugerie L, Seksik P, Nion-Larmurier I, et al. Predictors of Crohn's disease. Gastroenterology 2006;130(3):650–6.

17. Alli-Akintade L, Pruthvi P, Hadi N, et al. Race and fistulizing perianal Crohn's disease. J Clin Gastroenterol 2015;49(3):e21–3.

18. Gelbmann CM, Rogler G, Gross V, et al. Prior bowel resections, perianal disease, and a high initial Crohn's disease activity index are associated with corticosteroid resistance in active Crohn's disease. Am J Gastroenterol 2002;97(6):1438–45.

19. Parks AG. Pathogenesis and treatment of fistuila-in-ano. Br Med J 1961;1(5224): 463–9. Available at: http://www.pubmedcentral.nih.gov/articlerender.fcgi?artid= 1953161&tool=pmcentrez&rendertype=abstract.

20. Hughes LE. Surgical pathology and management of anorectal Crohn's disease. J R Soc Med 1978;71(9):644–51. Available at: http://www.pubmedcentral.nih. gov/articlerender.fcgi?artid=1436266&tool=pmcentrez&rendertype=abstract.

21. Siegmund B, Feakins RM, Bamias G, et al. Results of the fifth scientific workshop of the ECCO (II): pathophysiology of perianal fistulising disease. J Crohns Colitis 2016;10:377–86.

22. Milligan E, Morgan C. Surgical anatomy of the anal canal with special reference to anorectal fistulae. Lancet 1934;224(5804):1150–6.

23. Parks AG, Gordon PH, Hardcastle JD. A classification of fistula-in-ano. Br J Surg 1976;63(1):1–12.

24. Sandborn WJ, Fazio VW, Feagan BG, et al. AGA technical review on Perianal Crohn's disease. Gastroenterology 2003;125(5):1508–30.

25. Allan A, Keighley MRB, Hospital TG, et al. Management of perianal Crohn's disease. World J Surg 1988;12:198–202.

26. Williamson PR, Hellinger MD, Larach SW, et al. Twenty-year review of the surgical management of perianal Crohn's disease. Dis Colon Rectum 1995;38(4):389–92.

27. Michelassi F, Melis M, Rubin M, et al. Surgical treatment of anorectal complications in Crohn's disease. Surgery 2000;128(4):597–603.

28. Van Beers B, Grandlin C, Kartheuser A, et al. MRI of complicated anal fistulae: comparison with digital examination. J Comput Assist Tomogr 1994;18(1):87–90.

29. Wise PE, Schwartz DA. The evaluation and treatment of Crohn perianal fistulae: EUA, EUS, MRI, and other imaging modalities. Gastroenterol Clin North Am 2012;41(2):379–91.

30. Schwartz DA, Pemberton JH, Sandborn WJ. Diagnosis and treatment of perianal fistulas in Crohn disease. Ann Intern Med 2001;135:906–18.

31. Haggett PJ, Moore NR, Shearman JD, et al. Pelvic and perineal complications of Crohn's disease: assessment using magnetic resonance imaging. Gut 1995; 36(3):407–10. Available at: http://www.pubmedcentral.nih.gov/articlerender.fcgi? artid=1382455&tool=pmcentrez&rendertype=abstract.

32. Koelbel G, Schmiedl U, Majer MC, et al. Diagnosis of fistulae and sinus tracts in patients with Crohn disease: value of MR imaging. Am J Roentgenol 1989;152(5): 999–1003.

33. Mulder CJ, Wijers OB, Sars PR, et al. Endosonography of peri-anal and peri-colorectal fistula and/or abscess in Crohn's disease. Gastrointest Endosc 1990; 36(4):331–6.

34. Orsoni P, Barthet M, Portier F, et al. Prospective comparison of endosonography, magnetic resonance imaging and surgical findings in anorectal fistula and abscess complicating Crohn's disease. Br J Surg 1999;86(3):360–4.

35. Schwartz DA, Wiersema MJ, Dudiak KM, et al. A comparison of endoscopic ultrasound, magnetic resonance imaging, and exam under anesthesia for evaluation of Crohn's perianal fistulas. Gastroenterology 2001;121(5):1064–72.

36. Spradlin NM, Wise PE, Herline AJ, et al. A randomized prospective trial of endoscopic ultrasound to guide combination medical and surgical treatment for Crohn's perianal fistulas. Am J Gastroenterol 2008;103(10):2527–35.

37. Lahat A, Assulin Y, Beer-Gabel M, et al. Endoscopic ultrasound for perianal Crohn's disease: disease and fistula characteristics, and impact on therapy. J Crohns Colitis 2012;6(3):311–6.

38. Gecse KB, Bemelman W, Kamm MA, et al. A global consensus on the classification, diagnosis and multidisciplinary treatment of perianal fistulising Crohn's disease. Gut 2014;63(9):1381–92.

39. Schwartz DA, Ghazi LJ, Regueiro M, et al. Guidelines for the multidisciplinary management of Crohn's perianal fistulas. Inflamm Bowel Dis 2015;21(4):723–30.

40. Allan R, Cooke T. Evaluation of metronidazole in the management of Crohn's disease. Gut 1977;18:398–528.

41. Bernstein LH, Frank MS, Brandt LJ, et al. Healing of perineal Crohn's disease with metronidazole. Gastroenterology 1980;79(2):357–65.

42. Thia KT, Mahadevan U, Feagan BG, et al. Ciprofloxacin or metronidazole for the treatment of perianal fistulas in patients with Crohn's disease: a randomized, double-blind, placebo-controlled pilot study. Inflamm Bowel Dis 2009;15(1):17–24.

43. Dewint P, Hansen BE, Verhey E, et al. Adalimumab combined with ciprofloxacin is superior to adalimumab monotherapy in perianal fistula closure in Crohn's disease: a randomised, double-blind, placebo controlled trial (ADAFI). Gut 2014; 63(2):292–9.

44. Pearson DC, May GR, Fick GH, et al. Azathioprine and 6-mercaptopurine in Crohn disease: a meta-analysis. Ann Intern Med 1995;123:132–42.

45. Dejaco C, Harrer M, Waldhoer T, et al. Antibiotics and azathioprine for the treatment of perianal fistulas in Crohn's disease. Aliment Pharmacol Ther 2003; 18(11–12):1113–20.

46. Mahadevan U, Marion JF, Present DH. Fistula response to methotrexate in Crohn's disease: a case series. Aliment Pharmacol Ther 2003;1003–8. http://dx.doi.org/10.1046/j.0269-2813.2003.01790.x.

47. Lowry PW, Weaver AL, Tremaine WJ, et al. Combination therapy with oral tacrolimus (FK506) and azathioprine or 6-mercaptopurine for treatment-refractory Crohn's disease perianal fistulae. Inflamm Bowel Dis 1999;5(4):239–45. Available at: http://www.ncbi.nlm.nih.gov/pubmed/10579116.

48. Sandborn WJ, Present DH, Isaacs KL, et al. Tacrolimus for the treatment of fistulas in patients with Crohn's disease: a randomized, placebo-controlled trial. Gastroenterology 2003;125(2):380–8.

49. Hart AL, Plamondon S, Kamm MA. Topical tacrolimus in the treatment of perianal Crohn's disease: exploratory randomized controlled trial. Inflamm Bowel Dis 2007;13(3):245–53.

50. Present DH, Rutgeerts P, Targan S, et al. Infliximab for the treatment of fistulas in patients with Crohn's disease. N Engl J Med 1999;340(18):1398–405.

51. Sands BE, Anderson FH, Bernstein CN, et al. Infliximab maintenance therapy for fistulizing Crohn's disease. N Engl J Med 2004;350(9):876–85.

52. Lichtenstein GR, Yan S, Bala M, et al. Infliximab maintenance treatment reduces hospitalizations, surgeries, and procedures in fistulizing Crohn's disease. Gastroenterology 2005;128(4):862–9.

53. Colombel JF, Sandborn WJ, Rutgeerts P, et al. Adalimumab for maintenance of clinical response and remission in patients with Crohn's disease: the CHARM trial. Gastroenterology 2007;132(1):52–65.

54. Colombel J-F, Schwartz DA, Sandborn W, et al. Adalimumab for the treatment of fistulas in patients with Crohn's disease. Gut 2009;58:940–8.

55. Schreiber S, Lawrance IC, Thomsen O, et al. Randomised clinical trial: certolizumab pegol for fistulas in Crohn's disease: subgroup results from a placebo-controlled study. Aliment Pharmacol Ther 2011;33(2):185–93.

56. Sandborn WJ, Feagan BG, Rutgeerts P, et al. Vedolizumab as induction and maintenance therapy for Crohn's disease. N Engl J Med 2013;369(8):711–21.

57. Cohen Z. An approach to perirectal disease in inflammatory bowel disease. Inflamm Bowel Dis 1999;5(3):228–30.

58. Regueiro M, Mardini H. Treatment of perianal fistulizing Crohn's disease with infliximab alone or as an adjunct to exam under anesthesia with seton placement. Inflamm Bowel Dis 2003;9(2):98–103.

59. Topstad DR, Panaccione R, Heine JA, et al. Combined seton placement, infliximab infusion, and maintenance immunosuppressives improve healing rate in fistulizing anorectal Crohn's disease: a single center experience. Dis Colon Rectum 2003;46(5):577–83.

60. Rutgeerts P. Review article: treatment of perianal fistulizing Crohn's disease. Aliment Pharmacol Ther 2004;20(Suppl 4):106–10.

61. Yassin NA, Askari A, Warusavitarne J, et al. Systematic review: the combined surgical and medical treatment of fistulising perianal Crohn's disease. Aliment Pharmacol Ther 2014;40:741–9.

62. Balzola F, Bernstein C, Ho GT, et al. Fibrin glue is effective healing perianal fistulas in patients with Crohn's disease: commentary. Inflamm Bowel Dis Monit 2010;11(2):80–1.

63. Molendijk I, Bonsing BA, Roelofs H, et al. Allogeneic bone marrow-derived mesenchymal stromal cells promote healing of refractory perianal fistulas in patients with Crohn's disease. Gastroenterology 2015;149(4):918–27.e6.

64. Garcia-Olmo D, Schwartz DA. Cumulative evidence that mesenchymal stem cells promote healing of perianal fistulas of patients with Crohn's disease: going from bench to bedside. Gastroenterology 2015;149(4):853–7.

Endoscopic Delivery of Fecal Biotherapy in Inflammatory Bowel Disease

 CrossMark

David H. Kerman, MD

KEYWORDS

- Fecal Microbial Transplant (FMT) • Inflammatory Bowel Disease (IBD) • Dysbiosis
- Microbiome • Recurrent Clostridium Difficile Infection (RCDI)

KEY POINTS

- The intestinal microbiome plays an important role in the pathogenesis of dysbiotic conditions, namely in inflammatory bowel disease (IBD).
- Fecal microbiota transplantation (FMT) has been shown to be efficacious in restoring a dysbiotic state in recurrent *Clostridium difficile* infection (RCDI) with use of upper gastrointestinal (GI), lower GI, or encapsulated stool product.
- There is tremendous excitement in our ability to manipulate dysbiosis in IBD with utilization of FMT, but it is currently not allowable for therapeutic purposes of IBD without a proper approval with Investigational New Drug application through the Food and Drug Administration.
- Further research with proper regulatory oversight is required to enhance our knowledge of the safety and efficacy of FMT in IBD.

INTRODUCTION

The intestinal microbiota has been shown to play an important role in several gastrointestinal (GI) disorders, including inflammatory bowel disease (IBD). Evidence supporting the role of bacterial flora in IBD includes the use of antibiotics targeting enteric flora in prevention of postoperative recurrence of Crohn's disease (CD).[1] As our understanding of what constitutes imbalances of the intestinal microbiota expands, we are able to treat to target for a more "harmonious" balance. One unique example of this manipulation is the use of fecal microbial transplantation (FMT) for treatment of recurrent *Clostridium difficile* colitis (RCDI). FMT has been used since the fourth century in China, and was first reported in the medical literature when Eiseman and colleagues[2] used fecal enemas in 4 patients for treatment of pseudomembranous colitis. The past decade has seen a steep rise in the incidence of RCDI,[3] bringing FMT to the forefront of both scientific communities and the lay public. Success of FMT in RCDI has been shown by retrospective

Gastroenterology Fellowship Program, Division of Gastroenterology, University of Miami Miller School of Medicine, 1120 Northwest 14th Street, Suite 974, Miami, FL 33136, USA
E-mail address: dkerman@med.miami.edu

Gastrointest Endoscopy Clin N Am 26 (2016) 707–717
http://dx.doi.org/10.1016/j.giec.2016.06.006
1052-5157/16/© 2016 Elsevier Inc. All rights reserved.

reviews[4] and more recently by randomized controlled trials.[5] RCDI is prevalent in patients with IBD and also is a risk factor for negative outcomes. FMT use in the IBD population for RCDI has been shown to be both safe and efficacious.[6] The use of FMT to directly treat IBD, however, has shown mixed results. Given our ability to target the dysbiotic state with FMT, its use as targeted therapy has tremendous potential. Studies have involved a multidisciplinary approach, including gastroenterologists, infectious disease specialists, microbiologists, and patient volunteers. This overview discusses the practical considerations of FMT therapy with respect to our current understanding of safety and efficacy in IBD, screening for donors and recipients, specimen handling and storage, methods of delivery, and regulatory considerations.

REGULATORY GUIDELINES

Therapeutic use of FMT has not followed a traditional path toward investigation and approval. Practitioners in infectious disease and gastroenterology have used it in various forms for many years without formal regulatory guidelines, unprecedented for a biological product. Medical therapy centers presented early options for patients to undergo a therapeutic FMT procedure for indications such as obesity, irritable bowel syndrome, or IBD without regulatory oversight. These practices were primarily based on positive case series, although efficacy and safety were not entirely known. This changed in 2013 when the US Food and Drug Administration (FDA) announced that any practitioner who wished to perform FMT obtain approval through application for an Investigational New Drug (IND). This was subsequently amended to state that an FMT is allowable without an IND for the indication of RCDI only. All other indications would require an IND. It is important for practitioners to recognize that FMT has yet to fully be studied beyond the phase 1 and early phase 2 portions of drug approval. At the time of this publication, FMT is *not* allowable for therapeutic use in IBD unless an IND has been obtained. The most recent FDA draft guidance was issued in March of 2016.[7] This states that practitioners can use FMT for CDI not responding to standard therapies as long as full informed consent is obtained including the knowledge that FMT is an investigational therapy along with discussion of its reasonable foreseeable risks. The guidance mentions use of stool banks to obtain donor specimens and the regulatory oversight required when banks are used. It should be noted that the FDA is not changing its policy on enforcement discretion that allows for use of FMT without IND as long as

1. Full informed consent is obtained from the recipient that includes knowledge that FMT is an experimental treatment.
2. The stool is not obtained from a stool bank.
3. A licensed health care provider tests the donor's blood and stool for the purposes of FMT.

At of the time of this draft, the regulation is up for public discussion on the FDA Web site. Key issues are defining what constitutes a stool bank and how to regulate their distribution of FMT product, particularly across state lines.

DONOR AND RECIPIENT CONSIDERATIONS

Excitement within the scientific community over the therapeutic potential of FMT has translated to the lay public. Despite the apparent "ick factor" of the procedure, patients with IBD have demonstrated a willingness to undergo FMT, especially among those with more severe disease.[8] Despite this willingness to undergo the procedure, many patients still find it difficult to seek out a suitable donor. There is also tremendous expense involved with the process of FMT, as many insurance carriers will not pay for the screening tests needed on both stool and serum for a healthy donor. The time involved to process the screening tests for the donor can lead to delays and further morbidity with the anticipated recipient.

An FMT donor for the purpose of IBD should be relatively healthy and free of diseases associated with intestinal microbiota (**Box 1**). Food allergies of the recipient should be taken into consideration when assessing the appropriate donor to prevent allergic complications following transplantation. Initially in RCDI, the FDA wanted recipients to know their donors, but this came with many practical barriers. There are theoretic advantages and disadvantages for the recipient to have a familiar relationship to the donor. A first-degree relative may share genetic likeness that could confer a higher probability of successful engraftment. Alternatively, this shared genetic profile in IBD may prove an unhealthy match for treating a genetically based inflammatory disorder in the host. One possible disadvantage of using an intimate contact from the same household is the possible shared microbial environment that led to an inflammatory state in the first place. We may find that unrelated donors allow for implantation of a richer diversity in intestinal flora when compared with related donors. Ethical questions also present themselves when relatives serve as donors in the event that an adverse event may occur. A central stool bank that uses anonymous donations would avert awkward encounters during those instances.

For the purpose of informed consent, a donor must be at least 18 years of age. If younger than 18, both child and parental consent must be obtained. Donor selection should include the same screening process that is required for blood donation. A joint society letter from the Infectious Disease Society of America (IDSA), American Society for Gastrointestinal Endoscopy (ASGE), American College of Gastroenterology (ACG), the North American Society for Pediatric Gastroenterology, Hepatology, and Nutrition (NASPGHN), and the American Gastroenterological Association (AGA) written to the FDA provides a consensus guidance on donor selection and stool testing for the purposes of FMT for RCDI.[9] This document includes a reference to the AABB Donor Questionnaire Documents on the FDA biologics Web site. These requirements are for minimum safety purposes and should be followed for IBD. Beyond these minimum safety precautions, we do not know what donor considerations should be used. The

---

Box 1
Minimum required serum and stool testing before performing fecal microbial transplantation (FMT)

Serum Testing (within 4 weeks of FMT)
   HAV-immunoglobulin M
   HBsAg
   Anti-HCV ab
   Human immunodeficiency virus–EIA
   RPR

Stool testing (within 4 weeks of FMT)
   Clostridium difficile toxin B (preferably polymerase chain reaction)
   Culture for enteric pathogens
   Ova and parasites (if travel hx suggests)

Abbreviations: EIA, enzyme immunoassay; HAV, hepatitis A virus; HBsAg, hepatitis B surface antigen; HCV ab, hepatitis C virus antibody; hx, history; RPR, rapid plasma reagin.

following are the exclusion criteria that are recommended by the consensus guidance statement:

Exclusion Criteria

- A history of antibiotic treatment during the preceding 3 months of donation
- A history of intrinsic GI illness, including IBD, irritable bowel syndrome, GI malignancies, or major GI surgical procedures
- A history of autoimmune or atopic illness or ongoing immune modulating therapy
- A history of chronic pain syndromes (fibromyalgia, chronic fatigue) or neurologic, neurodevelopmental disorders
- Metabolic syndrome, obesity (body mass index of >30), or moderate-to-severe undernutrition (malnutrition)
- A history of malignant illnesses or ongoing oncologic therapy

In our practice for RCDI, we offer the options for the patient to find a donor with the preceding criteria and then have the donor undergo appropriate stool and blood screening tests. We also offer a third-party option of a prescreened, frozen, stored FMT product that has IND approval at a low-cost option. Invariably, patients prefer the route of the third-party purchase for their procedure to avoid treatment delays. Additionally, this allows patients to avoid awkward encounters with friends or relatives who may feel uncomfortable with the process altogether. Moving forward, there should be standardization of donor recruitment along with better understanding of how to match donor to recipient, as well as predictive factors in the recipients and donors that may increase the likelihood of success with FMT.

PUBLISHED EFFICACY DATA OF FECAL MICROBIOTA TRANSPLANTATION IN INFLAMMATORY BOWEL DISEASE

Therapeutic challenges in IBD persist despite the advent of newer molecular targets in biological therapy. With our current toolkit, clinicians still face the unenviable task of informing patients with IBD that the overall response rate to current therapeutic modalities reaches only 50%. In the past 5 years, FMT has emerged as a window into the science of manipulation of dysbiosis. As such, the number of studies investigating the utility of FMT as a viable treatment option for a dysbiotic state has risen exponentially.[10] Our understanding of what constitutes a healthy microbiota is evolving. From a bird's-eye perspective, reduced diversity of flora is seen in patients with IBD when compared with healthy controls.[11] There are also differences in both the type and function of flora that are present in patients with IBD. Dysbiosis is characterized by decreased *firmacutes* and *bacteroides* and an increase in *proteobacteria* and *actinobacteria*.[11] Antibiotics have been shown to ameliorate both small intestinal bacterial overgrowth (SIBO)[12] and pouchitis,[13] and smaller studies have shown their ability to induce remission in a small trial in *C difficile* (CD).[14] FMT offers the theoretic advantage over antibiotics of restoring diversity of flora to potentially cure a dysbiotic state.

The efficacy of therapeutic use of FMT for IBD has yet to be determined, as results of both case reports and clinical trials have been mixed. The first case report of FMT in IBD was a physician who used a 1-time FMT via enema to achieve both endoscopic and histologic remission 6 months following the intervention.[15] Thomas Borody has been performing and studying FMT for many years. These have been performed in Australia where regulatory agencies have not provided restrictions on its use. A large series of case reports provided mostly positive results, but they lacked controls and were open-labeled.[16,17] Additionally, the cases varied with regard to route of administration, preparation of the stool product, and screening protocol. Successful open-labeled trials have been shown in the pediatric population in CD.[18] A recent systematic review and meta-analysis of FMT in IBD included 18 studies with only 1 randomized controlled trial (RCT).[19] This found an overall remission rate of 45%, which decreased to 36% when evaluating cohort studies only. When accounting for FMT done for ulcerative colitis (UC), the remission rate dipped to 22%.

Three RCTs recently published have only somewhat enhanced our understanding, although again with variable outcomes. In the trial by Moayyedi and colleagues,[20] patients were randomized to receive either weekly fecal enemas or water enemas for 6 weeks with the primary outcome measure of remission of UC. Use of immune suppressive therapy, including anti–tumor necrosis factor (anti-TNF), agents was permitted in the study. The data safety monitoring board (DSMB) stopped the trial early after only 4 of the 27 patients were in remission in the FMT arm, and 2 of the 26 patients in the placebo arm, citing low likelihood of achieving their primary outcome measure. After this occurred, patients already screened and enrolled were allowed to continue with the treatments. Notably, these patients received FMT from one specific donor (donor B) and had a high response rate, pushing the results into clinical significance (9/38 [24%] FMT patients achieved remission versus 2/37 [5%] in the placebo group). Despite a small sample size, this was the largest RCT for FMT in UC. Two interesting findings emerged from this study. First, patients who underwent FMT had a statistically significant increase in microbial diversity when compared with the placebo group at week 6. These patients also had a significant effect of similar fecal microbial profile to their donors. Second, the study used 6 donors; with patients treated by one specific donor (donor B) conferring a positive effect for 7 of 11 patients receiving this stool, although without achieving significance versus placebo. Other researchers have posited that the diversity of donor flora can influence the success of FMT for IBD. [21] Although this is an intriguing finding, further research is required before fully understanding what donor or stool profile will be beneficial to which recipient.

In the trial by Rossen and colleagues,[22] patients with UC were randomized to receive FMT via nasogastric tube (NGT) from healthy donors or given autologous fecal material with primary endpoint of clinical remission at week 12. The intervention was performed at the beginning of the trial and again 3 weeks later. Notably, patients who had received anti-TNF or methotrexate within 8 weeks of the trial were excluded. An interim analysis by the DSMB also advised termination of the trial after 48 patients were recruited due to futility. At 12 weeks, 7 (30%) of 23 patients receiving FMT from donors achieved clinical remission versus 8 (32%) of 25 in the autologous FMT group. Stool analysis revealed changes in the responders to donated FMT had a microbial profile similar toward those of their donors. The authors posited route of administration and need for increased number of FMT procedures as a reason for lack of more robust response in the donated FMT group.

Most recently, a multicenter RCT performed in Australia by Paramsothy and colleagues[23] compared participants who underwent a single FMT delivered via colonoscopy, then 5 FMT enemas per week for a total of 8 weeks with those receiving placebo enemas (matched for color and smell). The investigators showed a trend toward significant differences in both steroid-free and endoscopic remission and response rates between the groups. This intensive therapy used pooled donors to negate any potential influence of a single donor and found a large increase in fecal diversity in the successfully treated patients.

The aforementioned RCTs represent a positive step forward toward our understanding of how IBD responds to manipulation of the intestinal microbiota. There are currently more than 35 registered trials on clinicaltrials.gov that involve FMT as therapy for IBD. Progress in our ability and understanding will require more standardized methods with randomization to safely and reasonably use FMT as a clinical therapeutic for IBD. Specific questions must include microbial analysis to appreciate the specific donor and recipient profiles that are required for clinical success.

PUBLISHED SAFETY DATA OF FECAL MICROBIOTA TRANSPLANTATION FOR INFLAMMATORY BOWEL DISEASE

Safety data for FMT are limited given the lack of long-term data. Most data are derived from small case series and retrospective data in patients with RCDI. Normally, the FDA would require a biological product to undergo safety and efficacy studies in the preclinical and phase 1 to 3 trials. With FMT, initial safety and efficacy data have come from publication of retrospective clinical reports and cohort studies. More rigorous controlled trials are only now emerging[5] and have shed light on more accurate safety and efficacy data. In RCDI, FMT appears to be relatively safe in the short term based on these. Long-term data, however, are lacking and our understanding of what can be transferred via the intestinal microbiota is mainly speculative with regard to what can be transferred from one person's microbial population to another's (**Box 2**).

Safety data specific to FMT for IBD is from the cohort series mentioned previously, the 2 RCTs, and a multicenter retrospective series. The procedure is generally well tolerated with few adverse side effects; however, follow-up is variable among the trials noted. In the systematic review and meta-analysis, minor events, such as fever, elevation of C-reactive protein, increased stool frequency, and abdominal bloating, were noted. Most of the adverse events could be attributed to use of NGT, and all were self-limited from 1 to 3 days post-FMT. In the trial of Moayyedi and colleagues,[20] 5 adverse events were noted, with one flare of UC 3 weeks into the trial requiring urgent colectomy. Three others (2 from the FMT and 1 in placebo arm) developed infectious complications that resolved with antibiotics. In the trial by Rossen and colleagues[22] administered via NGT, most patients had minor self-limited adverse events such as borborygmus and increased stool frequency and there were no reported infectious complications. One patient was later discovered to have CD after a small bowel perforation that occurred

---

Box 2
Adverse events

Short-term minor adverse events

- Abdominal discomfort
- Bloating
- Flatulence
- Diarrhea
- Borborygmus
- Vomiting
- Transient fever

Potential long-term adverse events

- Infection (recognized and unrecognized)
- Alterations in microbiota and risk of disease:
  - Obesity
  - Diabetes mellitus
  - Inflammatory bowel disease
  - Colon cancer

5 weeks after the FMT. Another patient developed severe infection related to cytomegalovirus (CMV), but was noted to be in the autologous FMT arm of the trial.

Colleen Kelly and colleagues[6] performed a multicenter retrospective series of immunocompromised patients who underwent FMT for RCDI. This analysis included 36 patients who were considered immunocompromised due to their IBD medication. Of these patients, 16 were on anti-TNF agents, and 2 were on alpha-4 integrin inhibition. Three patients with UC ended up with colectomy, but none of these surgeries were related to the FMT. One patient underwent colectomy within 1 month of the procedure, but had worsening IBD before the FMT. The other 2 patients underwent colectomy more than 100 days following the FMT. As with other studies, nausea, bloating, and discomfort were common and occurred in patients with IBD with similar frequency as other immunocompromised patients in the study.

Case reports are emerging of FMT causing flare of patients IBD. The trial by Moayyedi and colleagues[20] previously described highlights one such case. Another in the records of Massachusetts General Hospital was of a CMV infection following a 37-year-old man who performed home FMT enemas without physician guidance.[24] A second case of UC flare in a man with previously quiescent colitis was reported following FMT for RCDI.[25] One trial of FMT for UC with 5 adult patients resulted in transient elevation of C-reactive protein in all subjects following the procedure.[26] Caution should be used when considering FMT in patients with IBD given these reports.

FECAL MATERIAL PREPARATION AND STORAGE

Before our use of a third-party FMT product, our practice used a patient-recruited donor to provide a stool specimen on the day of the procedure; preferably within 4 to 6 hours and brought in a cooler with an ice pack. Patients would also provide a blender for homogenization of the material. There has been no standardized protocol for preparation of donor stool, and reports vary as to the amount of stool required to blend (anywhere from 50–300 g in 300–500 mL of diluent). Distilled water, normal saline, or milk has been used as diluent for mixing stool, but no single substance has been shown to be more effective. The mixture can then be poured over a coffee filter or gauze pad to filter any particulate matter that is likely not useful for transfer and can interfere with the procedure. There are obvious aesthetic and infection control challenges to this aforementioned process. Our hospital uses a terminal cleaning of the endoscopy suite any time FMT is performed so as to minimize infection risk.

A recent randomized trial of 219 patients with RCDI compared use of fresh stool versus frozen prepared stool via enema.[27] The investigators found that use of the frozen stool product was noninferior to use of fresh stool. An open-labeled feasibility study of encapsulated frozen stool product delivered via oral administration was studied in 20 patients with RCDI.[28] The investigators observed no serious adverse events in their study along with an initial cure of RCDI in 14 (70%) of 20 patients. Retreatment of the 6 failures obtained resolution of diarrhea in another 4 patients. These trials demonstrate the feasibility, safety, and efficacy of a prepared, frozen product that can be immediately used in patients with RCDI. The FDA is working closely with investigators to ensure standardization of material processing is established, and the process for a centralized stool bank may fall under the auspice of Current Good Manufacturing Practices (CGMPs) as with other pharmaceutical products.[29]

Suggested storage of a frozen FMT product should be in a −20°C freezer and should not be kept for longer than a 6-month time period. Thawing of the product should take place 1 hour before infusion with use of warm water or 4 hours prior at room temperature. Once a product is thawed, it should not be refrozen.[30]

PATIENT PREPARATION

The most important factor in success of FMT engraftment in patients is the cessation of antibiotics 24 to 48 hours before the procedure. Use of antibiotics within 30 days of intervention was part of the exclusion criteria in the trials of FMT for IBD.

Most trials for RCDI made use of a bowel lavage before the infusion of FMT product, but there are no data to suggest that this is necessary for success of the FMT. Bowel lavage has been shown to have a lasting effect on healthy individuals,[31] and the only 2 RCTs of FMT for IBD differed in their use of lavage before intervention. In IBD, the effect of the bowel lavage is not known.

When infusing FMT via the upper GI route, it is important to use both a proton pump inhibitor and antiemetic medication before and after the procedure to minimize risk of aspiration. Patients undergoing FMT via lower GI route should use loperamide or an antidiarrheal equivalent before and after the procedure to ensure adequate time of retention.

METHODS OF DELIVERY

Practitioners have the various options of delivery method for the FMT product (**Table 1**). There is no consensus on which delivery method is preferred. For both upper GI and lower GI delivery methods, a standard 60-mL syringe is used to directly deliver the FMT product via nasogastric tube or the therapeutic channel through the endoscope. In the review of FMT for IBD by Coleman and Rubin,[19] no single method of delivery demonstrated superiority, although the study was not designed as a comparative analysis. In a systematic review and meta-analysis of 273 patients undergoing FMT for RCDI, Kassam and colleagues[4] found that delivery via lower GI route led to a higher rate of clinical resolution when compared with upper GI delivery (91.4% vs 81.3%). Additionally, a recent collaborative analysis of 305 patients suggested a slight increased risk of clinical failure of FMT via the upper GI delivery method for RCDI versus lower GI delivery.[32] Small studies of frozen capsulized stool for RCDI were less effective than lower GI delivery, and also required multiple treatments.

Each method of delivery carries its own advantages and disadvantages. In IBD, a colonoscopy carries the added benefit of direct visualization of involved mucosa. In my practice, I prefer this method for patients with IBD with RCDI, as I can determine whether the mucosa has the appearance of an IBD flare or if pseudomembranes are present. Alternatively, FMT via enema carries a much lower risk profile given the decreased need for anesthesia. The upper GI approach appears safe in UC, but carries multiple risks for patients with CD. In a patient with proximal fibrostenotic disease, risk of partial small bowel obstruction or ileus is an absolute contraindication to use of the upper GI approach. Aspiration risk via this route is also a very real concern.

Table 1 Patient preparation and dose by delivery route					
Route of Administration	Dose of FMT	Bowel Lavage	Antibiotics	PPI	Loperamide
UGI via NGT or upper endoscopy	50 mL	+/−	NO	YES + anti-emetic	—
Lower enema	50–250 mL	+/−	NO	—	+/−
Lower colonoscopy	250 mL	YES	NO	—	YES

Abbreviations: FMT, fecal microbial transplantation; NGT, nasogastric tube; PPI, proton pump inhibitor; UGI, upper gastrointestinal.

FMT via enema, on the other hand, has a very low risk profile, but could be difficult for some patients to retain.

Dosage of the FMT product is also not known for IBD. In RCDI, FMT has been tremendously successful with 1-time dosing, and patients who recur tend to do well with a second treatment. In IBD, there is no such established record of success with any dosing regimen. There seems to be a need for repeated treatments based on a persistently dysbiotic state in these patients and from recent trials, but further RCTs on safety, efficacy, and dosing are necessary to determine adequate usage in IBD.

FUTURE DIRECTIONS

Manipulation of the intestinal microbiome remains a clinical and scientific challenge. Unfortunately, the success of FMT in RCDI has not been reproduced in IBD. The dysbiotic state in patients with IBD is clearly a more complex target to treat than in RCDI. Simple whole stool transplantation in its various iterations has shown some promise, but true safety and efficacy are not yet known. Rigorous controlled trials with long-term safety data paired with national registries that are able to store and characterize donor and recipient traits now and in the future are essential to answering innumerable questions for investigators. IBD is only one of a host of diseases affected by intestinal dysbiosis that FMT offers promising therapies. Future research should target specific microbial disturbances that match therapy to disease rather than use of blunt tool of FMT. FMT clearly plays a role in manipulating disease treatment and dysbiosis, but only through rigorous testing under oversight of regulatory agencies will the medical field be able to bring this important technique to clinical fruition.

REFERENCES

1. Rutgeerts P, Hiele M, Geboes K, et al. Controlled trial of metronidazole treatment for prevention of Crohn's recurrence after ileal resection. Gastroenterology 1995; 108(6):1617–21.
2. Eiseman B, Silen W, Bascom GS, et al. Fecal enema as an adjunct in the treatment of pseudomembranous enterocolitis. Surgery 1958;44(5):854–9.
3. Lessa FC, Mu Y, Bamberg WM, et al. Burden of *Clostridium difficile* infection in the United States. N Engl J Med 2015;372(9):825–34.
4. Kassam Z, Lee CH, Yuan Y, et al. Fecal microbiota transplantation for *Clostridium difficile* infection: systematic review and meta-analysis. Am J Gastroenterol 2013; 108(4):500–8.
5. van Nood E, Vrieze A, Nieuwdorp M, et al. Duodenal infusion of donor feces for recurrent *Clostridium difficile*. N Engl J Med 2013;368(5):407–15.
6. Kelly CR, Ihunnah C, Fischer M, et al. Fecal microbiota transplant for treatment of *Clostridium difficile* infection in immunocompromised patients. Am J Gastroenterol 2014;109(7):1065–71.
7. Transplantation To Treat Clostridium difficile Infection Not Responsive to Standard Therapies; Draft Guidance for Industry; Availability. Available at: https://www.federalregister.gov/articles/2016/03/01/2016-04372/enforcement-policy-regarding-investigational-new-drug-requirements-for-use-of-fecal-microbiota-for.
8. Kahn SA, Vachon A, Rodriquez D, et al. Patient perceptions of fecal microbiota transplantation for ulcerative colitis. Inflamm Bowel Dis 2013;19(7):1506–13.
9. FMT Joint Society Consensus Guidance. Available at: https://www.gastro.org/research/Joint_Society_FMT_Guidance.pdf.
10. Smith MB, Kelly C, Alm EJ. Policy: how to regulate faecal transplants. Nature 2014;506(7488):290–1.

11. Kostic AD, Xavier RJ, Gevers D. The microbiome in inflammatory bowel disease: current status and the future ahead. Gastroenterology 2014;146(6):1489–99.

12. Pimentel M. Review of rifaximin as treatment for SIBO and IBS. Expert Opin Investig Drugs 2009;18(3):349–58.

13. Shen B, Achkar JP, Lashner BA, et al. A randomized clinical trial of ciprofloxacin and metronidazole to treat acute pouchitis. Inflamm Bowel Dis 2001;7(4):301–5.

14. Prantera C, Lochs H, Campieri M, et al. Antibiotic treatment of Crohn's disease: results of a multicentre, double blind, randomized, placebo-controlled trial with rifaximin. Aliment Pharmacol Ther 2006;23(8):1117–25.

15. Bennet JD, Brinkman M. Treatment of ulcerative colitis by implantation of normal colonic flora. Lancet 1989;1(8630):164.

16. Borody TJ, George L, Andrews P, et al. Bowel-flora alteration: a potential cure for inflammatory bowel disease and irritable bowel syndrome? Med J Aust 1989; 150(10):604.

17. Borody TJ, Warren EF, Leis S, et al. Treatment of ulcerative colitis using fecal bacteriotherapy. J Clin Gastroenterol 2003;37:42–7.

18. Suskind DL, Brittnacher MJ, Wahbeh G, et al. Fecal microbial transplant effect on clinical outcomes and fecal microbiome in active Crohn's disease. Inflamm Bowel Dis 2015;21(3):556–63.

19. Coleman RJ, Rubin D. Fecal microbial transplantation as therapy for inflammatory bowel disease: a systematic review and meta-analysis. J Crohns Colitis 2014;8: 1569–81.

20. Moayyedi P, Surette MG, Kim PT, et al. Fecal microbiota transplantation induces remission in patients with active ulcerative colitis in a randomized controlled trial. Gastroenterology 2015;149(1):102–9.

21. Vermeire S, Joossens M, Verbeke K, et al. Donor species richness determines faecal microbiota transplantation success in inflammatory bowel disease. J Crohns Colitis 2016;10(4):387–94.

22. Rossen NG, Fuentes S, van der Spek MJ, et al. Findings from a randomized controlled trial of fecal transplantation for patients with ulcerative colitis. Gastroenterology 2015;149(1):110–8.

23. Paramsothy S, Kamm M, Walsh A, et al. Multi donor intense faecal microbiota transplantation is an effective treatment for resistant ulcerative colitis: a randomised placebo-controlled trial. Gastroenterology 2016;150(4):S122–3.

24. Hohmann EL, Ananthakrishnan AN, Deshpande V. Case records of the Massachusetts General Hospital. N Engl J Med 2014;371:668–75.

25. De Leon LM, Watson JB, Kelly CR. Transient flare of ulcerative colitis after fecal microbiota transplantation for recurrent *Clostridium difficile* infection. Clin Gastroenterol Hepatol 2013;11(8):1036–8.

26. Angelberger S, Reinisch W, Makristathis A, et al. Temporal bacterial community dynamics vary among ulcerative colitis patients after fecal microbiota transplantation. Am J Gastroenterol 2013;108(10):1620–30.

27. Lee CH, Steiner T, Petrof EO, et al. Frozen vs fresh fecal microbiota transplantation and clinical resolution of diarrhea in patients with recurrent *Clostridium difficile* infection: a randomized clinical trial. JAMA 2016;315(2):142–9.

28. Youngster I, Russell GH, Pindar C, et al. Oral, capsulized, frozen fecal microbiota transplantation for relapsing *Clostridium difficile* infection. JAMA 2014;312(17): 1772–8.

29. Khoruts A, Sadowsky MJ, Hamilton MJ. Development of fecal microbial transplantation suitable for mainstream medicine. Clin Gastroenterol Hepatol 2015; 13:246–50.

30. Openbiome.org Storage Controls and Materials Specifications. Available at: http://static1.squarespace.com/static/50e0c29ae4b0a05702af7e6a/t/56e9bbea 3c44d843bfbfb3f5/1458158571207/Storage+Controls+and+Material+Specifi cations+%281%29.pdf.
31. Drago L, Toscano M, De Grandi R, et al. Persisting changes of intestinal micro-biota after bowel lavage and colonoscopy. Eur J Gastroenterol Hepatol 2016; 28(5):532–7.
32. Furuya-Kanamori L, Doi SA, Paterson DL, et al. Upper versus lower GI delivery for transplantation of fecal microbiota in recurrent or refractory *Clostridium difficile* infection: a collaborative analysis of individual patient data from 14 studies. J Clin Gastroenterol 2016. p. 1–6.

Motility Evaluation in the Patient with Inflammatory Bowel Disease

Sherine M. Abdalla, MD[a], Gorav Kalra, MD[b],
Baha Moshiree, MD, MS-CI[c],*

KEYWORDS

- Functional bowel disease • Motility disorders • Gastroparesis
- Gastroesophageal reflux disease • Irritable bowel syndrome
- Dyssynergic defecation • Fecal incontinence • Small bowel bacterial overgrowth

KEY POINTS

- Patients with inflammatory bowel diseases (IBD) suffer frequently from functional bowel diseases (FBD) and motility disorders.
- Complete evaluation of ongoing symptoms not related to an inflammatory flare in patients with IBD should be prompt with consideration of these motility disorders for which diagnostic studies are now available.
- Management of FBD and motility disorders in IBD combined with continued treatment of a patient's IBD symptoms will likely lead to better clinical outcomes and improve the patient's quality of life.

INTRODUCTION

Patients with inflammatory bowel disease (IBD) have significantly higher rates of functional bowel diseases (FBD) as compared with healthy controls[1,2] and often require motility evaluation for ongoing symptoms not thought to be related to an IBD flare. In fact, 66% of patients with IBD in one study met Rome III criteria for at least one FBD and the number of FBD symptoms correlated positively with anxiety/depression scores and negatively with health-related quality-of-life scores.[1] Given the high

Disclosure Statement: Nothing to disclose (S.M. Abdalla and G. Kalra). Speaker for Medtronic, Grant Support: Prometheus Laboratory (B. Moshiree) (IRB # 20130535).
[a] Department of Medicine, Jackson Memorial Hospital, University of Miami Miller School of Medicine, 1611 NW 12th Avenue, Central Building, 600D, Miami, FL 33136, USA; [b] Department of Medicine, Jackson Memorial Hospital, University of Miami Miller School of Medicine, 1120 Northwest 14th Street, CRB, 11th Floor, Miami, FL 33136, USA; [c] Department of Medicine, University of Miami Miller School of Medicine, 1120 Northwest 14th Street, CRB Suite 971, Miami, FL 33136, USA
* Corresponding author.
E-mail address: bmoshiree@med.miami.edu

prevalence of motility disorders in patients with IBD resulting in diminished quality of life and sometimes narcotics use, it is important for physicians to recognize and treat comorbid motility disorders and FBD. The goals of this review were to summarize the most recent literature on motility disturbances in patients with IBD and to give a brief overview of the ranges of motility disturbances, from reflux disease to anorectal disorders, and discuss their diagnosis and specific management.

GASTROESOPHAGEAL REFLUX DISEASE IN INFLAMMATORY BOWEL DISEASE

Gastroesophageal reflux disease (GERD) is a widely spread condition, with a reported prevalence of up to 27.8% of the US population.[3] IBD and GERD share upper gastrointestinal (GI) symptoms, such as heartburn, chest pain, and regurgitation. In more advanced upper GI involvement in IBD, patients may even present with dysphagia, odynophagia, worsening reflux symptoms, or obstructive symptoms, such as early satiety, postprandial vomiting, and weight loss.[4] GERD is encountered more frequently in patients with IBD than in the general population. In one study of more than 450 patients with IBD, the prevalence of GERD was 62% in ulcerative colitis (UC) and 72% in Crohn's disease (CD), and having a diagnosis of GERD was associated with reduced quality of life.[2] Although the esophagus is the least common location to be affected by CD in the GI tract,[4] it is likely underdiagnosed in adults due to lack of endoscopic biopsies of the esophagus.[4] The involvement of upper GI tract in IBD is increasingly becoming recognized, however, due to the now more frequent utilization of upper GI endoscopy in the assessment of patients with IBD.

GERD can be diagnosed clinically by improvement of typical symptoms with proton pump inhibitor (PPI) therapy and/or endoscopically by an upper endoscopy with biopsies showing esophagitis, or objectively by measuring acidity and duration of acid reflux episodes using a 24-hour ambulatory esophageal pH monitoring system. The diagnosis of CD esophagitis is more challenging due to the similarity of its manifestations to those of more common entities (eg, GERD).[5]

The prevalence of esophageal CD ranges from 0.2% to 11.2% in adults and up to 43.0% in children.[6,7] The prevalence of macroscopic upper GI tract inflammation in CD on endoscopy ranges from 30% to 64% of patients with CD in pediatric literature,[8,9] whereas microscopic inflammation had been reported to be present in 70% of patients.[10,11] Consensus among gastroenterologists regarding the definition of what qualifies to be significant upper GI involvement in IBD is yet to be established.[12] Although most of the literature links upper GI tract involvement to CD, the once widespread notion that UC is never associated with upper GI tract involvement is no longer considered valid.[12] Albeit used to be considered a separate entity that may not coexist with more distal disease in the 1998 Vienna classification of IBD,[13] upper GI involvement in CD has been accepted to accompany distal disease in the 2005 Montreal classification of CD.[14]

Endoscopically, GERD esophagitis has 3 stages: active, healing, and scarring,[15,16] based on the degree of presence of redness, necrotic debris, regenerating epithelium, and epithelial staining with Lugol iodine. The endoscopic findings in CD esophagitis are similar to those of colonic disease, and usually manifest as areas of inflammation, linear ulcerations, or, in more advanced disease, mucosal nodularity, cobblestone appearance, fistulas, fibrosis, stenosis, and/or strictures.[4–6,17] Histologically, CD esophagitis shows segmental, focal inflammatory infiltration of the lamina propria, extending between the muscle fibers of the muscularis mucosa, consisting mainly of lymphocytes, and associated with edema, dilated lymphatics, and epithelioid granulomas in the lamina propria, and may be associated with focally enhanced gastritis.[17]

Granulomas are considered the histologic hallmark of CD of the esophagus, given that other causes of granulomatous inflammation of the GI are excluded and other manifestations of CD, such as colonic involvement and non-GI manifestations, are present.[17] On the other hand, GERD esophagitis has been associated with mostly nonspecific inflammatory changes,[16] including dilated intercellular spaces, intrapapillary blood vessel dilation, intraepithelial bleeding, elongated papillae, basal cell hyperplasia, acanthosis, intraepithelial eosinophils, and Langerhans cells. Granulomas should not be present in GERD-related esophagitis.

Given the potential histology differentiation of GERD and esophagitis due to CD, endoscopy with biopsy is indicated when even mild upper GI symptoms are present in patients already diagnosed with IBD.[4] However, because CD esophagitis may go undiagnosed or misdiagnosed in a subset of patients who are asymptomatic and as the correlation of upper GI symptoms with true endoscopically and pathologically proven disease in patients with CD has not been fully established, this warrants upper GI endoscopy in all patients with established CD. This differentiation between upper GI involvement in IBD and reflux esophagitis is important, as treatment modalities used to treat each entity are different and have long-term consequences.

PPIs are frequently used to manage the symptoms of GERD and for diagnosis of reflux. PPIs, however, also have anti-inflammatory properties with improvement of IBD itself, including a decreased risk of pouchitis after ileal pouch anal anastomosis (IPAA).[18] Lack of differentiation between the 2 entities usually results in inappropriate administration of PPI therapy for symptomatic relief, which although shown to be clinically beneficial in CD esophagitis by anecdotal reports,[19] has never been proven with high-quality-level evidence-based data.[20] PPI therapy, once started, is usually continued for prolonged periods of time and this may predispose patients to the long-term side effects, most notably vitamin B12 and iron deficiency, hypomagnesemia, and increased risk of osteoporosis, pathologic fractures, chronic kidney disease, pneumonia, and enteric infections,[21,22] especially because patients with CD are also at risk of malabsorption, *Clostridium difficile* infections, and fractures.[23,24] In this context, PPIs should perhaps be even avoided in patients with IBD because they further predispose to malnutrition and bacterial overgrowth syndrome,[25,26] which results in symptoms of nausea and bloating, further exacerbating patients' symptoms.

Our Recommendations

The authors therefore recommend routine upper GI endoscopy in all patients with IBD with biopsies performed in the upper and lower esophagus and, in particular, those with established or suspected CD with upper GI symptoms. Endoscopy may conveniently be performed at the time of colonoscopy especially in those with concomitant complaints of diarrhea, and may aid in identifying sites of unsuspected CD. Moreover, routine upper GI endoscopy may be considered a comprehensive evaluation tool for determining CD extent in patients with established CD, and allows for differentiation of UC from CD in patients with predominantly colonic involvement with no small bowel or patchy colonic involvement, which are both clear signs of CD.[12] Given the risks associated with PPI use, we recommend stepping down therapy when possible, as well as increased utilization of histamine receptor antagonists (H2RAs), such as ranitidine, and calcium-containing antacids for those with infrequent symptoms, as many patients with IBD are at risk for osteoporosis. In patients with atypical or extraesophageal GERD who lack typical symptoms of pyrosis and regurgitation, we recommend pH testing to avoid giving PPIs to patients without true GERD. Patients who do not have significant acid reflux on pH testing performed while off of PPI may be classified as having functional heartburn or reflux hypersensitivity, based on the presence or absence of symptom correlation to reflux events. Treatment of these patients is largely empiric, with trials of tricyclic antidepressants (TCAs), selective serotonin reuptake inhibitors (SSRIs), or gabapentin.[27] The authors also recommend avoidance of PPI therapy in patients with IBD, given the extensive long-term side effect profile of these agents, and the likely exacerbation of symptoms in these patients (**Fig. 1**).

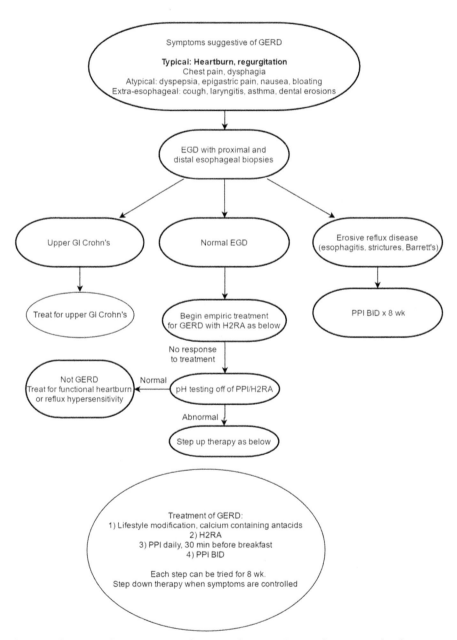

Fig. 1. Evaluation and management of suspected GERD. EGD, esophagogastroduodenoscopy.

GASTRIC DISORDERS IN INFLAMMATORY BOWEL DISEASE

Upper GI involvement occurs in approximately 34% of patients with CD, with the most common histologic correlates being gastric inflammation (84%), duodenal inflammation (28%), and gastric granulomas (23%).[28] Upper GI CD may be underdiagnosed, as a large proportion of these patients are asymptomatic.[29]

Gastroparesis

Gastroparesis (GP) is a syndrome of delayed gastric emptying in the absence of mechanical obstruction.[30] The cardinal symptoms include nausea and vomiting (N/V), early satiety, postprandial fullness, bloating, and upper abdominal pain. In severe cases, it can result in weight loss and malnutrition. The cause is most frequently idiopathic, although it can also result from diabetes, prior surgery, thyroid disease, neurologic disease, autoimmune disease, medications that retard gastric emptying, or following a viral illness.

Delayed gastric emptying (GE) appears to occur more frequently in patients with CD as compared with UC or healthy controls.[31,32] One study of children with IBD found that 33% of those with CD had had delayed GE, whereas all of the children with UC had normal GE.[31] After medical management of their CD and nutritional supplementation, significant improvements in GE were seen. Another study involving patients with IBD with moderate or no disease activity, 46% of patients with CD had prolonged GE, as compared with 20% of patients with UC.[32] In the subgroup of patients with CD, only vomiting was associated with delayed GE, whereas pain, nausea, bloating, and early satiety were not.

The mechanism for the delayed GE that occurs in some patients with IBD is unclear. In an animal model of rats with colitis induced via Trinitrobenzenesulfonic acid exposure, gastric emptying was found to be delayed, even in the absence of local gastric inflammation.[33] When these rats had their pelvic nerve sectioned, gastric emptying returned to baseline, suggesting that pelvic afferent nerve hyperactivity may contribute to delayed gastric emptying. Another study showed threefold elevations in postprandial cholecystokinin (CCK) levels in patients with CD versus controls, and postulated that excessive CCK release may contribute to delayed GE.[32] Other potential mechanisms could be loss of the interstitial cells of Cajal, which are lower in density in the small bowel tissue from patients with CD as compared with controls.[34]

Studies have also yielded conflicting results regarding the correlation between disease activity in CD and the presence of delayed GE. A study of 17 children with CD found that GE of solids was significantly slower in those who were malnourished, although liquid emptying was preserved, a phenomenon seen in patients with anorexia.[35] The delay in GE correlated with caloric intake and involvement of the duodenum (57%), but not with disease activity. Still, others have shown that disease activity may be correlated with prolonged GE.[36] Not surprisingly, patients with UC who have had previously undergone IPAA have similar solid-phase GE compared with controls,[37] but those with more than 6 bowel movements (BMs) per day have more rapid emptying of liquids as compared with those who had 6 or fewer BMs per day and those with constipation also have delayed GE.

Our Recommendations for Gastroparesis

An algorithm for the evaluation and management of suspected GP in patients with IBD is presented in **Fig. 2**. We recommend screening for delayed GE by solid-phase gastric emptying scintigraphy using the standardized method by Tougas and colleagues,[38] with a positive test having greater than 10% retention at 4 hours. Drugs that effect

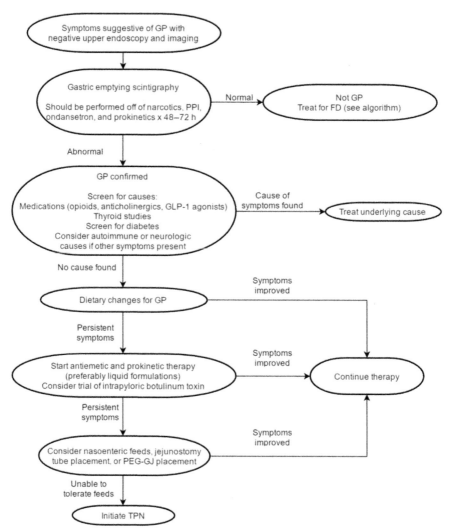

Fig. 2. Evaluation and management of suspected GP.

gastric motility, such as opioids, PPIs, ondansetron, prokinetics, anticholinergics, and glucagon-like peptide 1 (GLP-1) agonists, should be discontinued for 48 to 72 hours before testing. We recommend against the use of wireless motility capsule, as it is contraindicated in patients with CD given the risk of capsule retention in patients with possible strictures.[39] We also recommend against the use of 13-C breath testing, as its accuracy is contingent on normal small bowel absorption, which may not be the case in many patients with IBD. An upper endoscopy should be performed to exclude upper GI CD, other mucosal disease, celiac sprue, and mechanical obstruction.[30] In patients with CD, MRI enterography should be performed to exclude distal strictures resulting in recurrent partial small bowel obstruction that may mimic symptoms of GP. After GP is diagnosed, potential causes should be screened for and treated.

Initial management of gastroparesis consists of dietary modification with a low-fat, low insoluble fiber diet with small, frequent meals, and use of a liquid multivitamin.

Foods that have been found to provoke symptoms include those that are fatty, acidic, spicy, or contain significant roughage.[40] For those unable to tolerate solids, food can be blenderized or liquid nutritional supplements can be used. Antiemetics can be used to treat nausea. Although TCAs are widely used for GP, a multicenter trial of nortriptyline for idiopathic gastroparesis failed to show improvement over placebo.[41] Although macrolides are currently the most potent prokinetics available for treatment of GP,[42] their associated risk of developing *C difficile* infection with chronic use, risk of diarrhea, and potentially increased risk of sudden cardiac death limit their use in IBD.[43,44] Moreover, their long-term use is limited by the development of tachyphylaxis. As the only prokinetic approved by the Food and Drug Administration (FDA) for use in GP, metoclopramide is also to be avoided given the risk of irreversible tardive dyskinesia seen in less than 1% and inability to use the drug beyond 3 months,[45] but instead we favor the use of either domperidone, which requires an investigational new drug application through the FDA. Domperidone is a peripheral dopamine 2 (D2) receptor antagonist with effects similar to metoclopramide. It has been shown to be effective in diabetic GP,[46] although more rigorous trials are lacking. Domperidone can cause QT prolongation, and therefore electrocardiograms should be checked at baseline and while on therapy. Bethanechol is a muscarinic agonist that is inexpensive and sometimes used in the management of GP.[47] It increases lower esophageal sphincter (LES) tone and the amplitudes of gastric contractions, but does not accelerate GE.[48] Several newer prokinetics are being studied such as 5-HT$_4$ receptor agonists, including prucalopride and velusetrag, as well as ghrelin agonists and newer motilin agonists.[49] Relamorelin is a ghrelin agonist that has been shown to reduce vomiting frequency and accelerate gastric emptying in patients with diabetic GP.[50] When possible, liquid formulations of prokinetics should be used to facilitate absorption. **Table 1** summarizes the mechanism, dosing, and side effects of prokinetics.[30,45,47,48,51,52] We recommend against the use of gastric electrical stimulators in patients with IBD, as this has not been studied and given risk of theoretic autoimmune-type reaction to the pacer wires or infection risk in patients with IBD. In patients who are losing weight despite treatment for GP, we recommend nutritional supplementation via nasoenteric feeds, jejunostomy, or percutaneous endoscopic gastrojejunostomy (PEG-GJ) tube placement, or if these measures fail, start total parenteral nutrition.[30]

Functional Gastroduodenal Disorders

Functional gastroduodenal disorders are common in patients with IBD, with a prevalence of approximately 30%.[1] Based on the Rome IV criteria, these disorders are categorized into functional dyspepsia, belching disorders, chronic N/V disorders, and rumination syndrome.[53] Functional dyspepsia (FD) is defined as the presence of bothersome epigastric pain or burning, postprandial fullness, or early satiety, in the absence of the structural disease. Symptoms must be present for the past 3 months, with symptom onset at least 6 months before diagnosis. Patients with functional dyspepsia may be further classified as having postprandial distress syndrome (PDS), epigastric pain syndrome (EPS), or both. Patients with PDS have bothersome postprandial fullness or early satiety occurring at least 3 days per week, whereas those with EPS have bothersome epigastric pain or burning occurring at least 1 day per week. Heartburn is not considered a dyspeptic symptom, although it often coexists with FD. Although vomiting may be present in a subset of patients, it is uncommon in FD and its presence suggests another disorder, such as gastric outlet obstruction or GP. In addition to GP and upper GI CD, the differential diagnosis of FD includes GERD, peptic ulcer disease, *Helicobacter pylori*–associated dyspepsia, eosinophilic gastroenteritis, food allergies, and many others, including medications.[54] Medications

Table 1
Mechanism, dosing, and side effects of prokinetics

Drug	Mechanism	Physiologic Effect				Dose	Side Effects
		Anti-emetic	Effect on GE	Visceral Sensitivity	Antral Motility		
Metoclopramide	D2 antagonist 5-HT₄ agonist	+	↑	↓	↑	5–10 mg TID-QID Liquid preferred Intranasal: 10–20 mg TID	QT prolongation, extrapyramidal side effects (tardive dyskinesia <1%) Only FDA approved medication for GP Has a black-box warning
Domperidone	D2 antagonist (peripheral)	+	↑	↓		10–20 mg TID-QID	QT prolongation, Requires IND
Erythromycin	Motilin agonist		↑			40–250 mg TID Liquid preferred	QT prolongation, risk of C diff, efficacy limited by tachyphylaxis
Azithromycin	Motilin agonist		↑			Liquid: 200–400 mg daily in 5–10 mL IV: 250–500 mg daily	QT prolongation, risk of C diff, efficacy limited by tachyphylaxis
Bethanechol	Muscarinic agonist	−	No effect		↑	10–25 mg QID	Flushing, hypotension, bladder spasms
Prucalopride	5-HT₄ agonist		↑		↑	2–4 mg daily	Diarrhea

Abbreviations: 5-HT₄, 5-hydroxytryptamine receptor 4; C diff, *Clostridium difficile*, D2, dopamine receptor 2, FDA, Food and Drug Administration; GP, gastroparesis; IND, investigational new drug application; IV, intravenous; QID, 4 times a day; TID, 3 times a day; ↓, decreases; ↑, increases; +, present; −, not present.
Data from Refs.[30,45,47,48,51,52]

that have been implicated include nonsteroidal anti-inflammatory drugs, iron, calcium channel blockers, angiotensin-converting enzyme inhibitors, steroids, and methylxanthines, which include theophylline, pentoxifylline, and caffeine.

Our Recommendations for Functional Dyspepsia

An approach to the evaluation and management of FD is presented in **Fig. 3**. We recommend screening for and treating comorbid psychiatric illness, as dyspepsia is frequently associated with major depression and generalized anxiety disorder.[55]

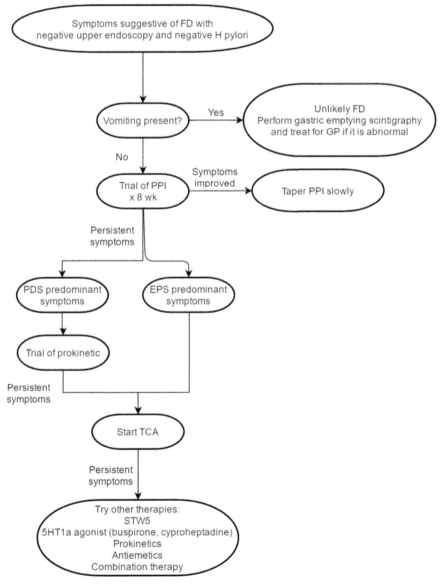

Fig. 3. Evaluation and management of FD.

Moreover, patients with IBD have higher rates of depression than the general popula-tion.[56] Initial management of FD includes testing and treating for *H pylori* as well as a trial of PPI. In patients who respond to a trial of PPI, we recommend step-down ther-apy to H2RAs, given the risks of PPI use in patients with IBD. For patients who meet criteria for PDS, a trial of a prokinetic should be considered. TCAs, such as amitripty-line, have been shown to be effective in FD, whereas SSRIs have not been effective.[57] STW 5 is a preparation of 9 herbs that has been shown to be safe and effective for the treatment of FD.[58] A trial of cyproheptadine can be considered, as it has been shown to reduce dyspeptic symptoms in children.[59] Buspirone, a $5-HT_{1A}$ agonist, causes fundic relaxation and has been shown to be effective in a small trial.[60]

PRESENCE OF IRRITABLE BOWEL SYNDROME IN INFLAMMATORY BOWEL DISEASE

Patients with IBD often present with multiple GI symptoms, such as mild to moderate diffuse or localized abdominal pain and diarrhea with increased fecal frequency and urgency, as seen in patients with FBD called irritable bowel syndrome with diarrhea (IBS-D). IBS-D is now better defined by the new Rome IV criteria as a bowel disorder with the omission of the word "functional," given the complex mechanisms involved in its pathogenesis combining genetic, environmental, psychological, and immunologic mechanisms, which then result in altered GI motility, visceral hypersensitivity with dis-turbances in brain-gut interactions, intestinal dysbiosis, and immune activation similar to IBD.[61] In fact, a significant portion of patients with IBD, a third of patients with UC, and half of patients with CD, continue to have abdominal pain while in remission confirmed by the lack of any inflammatory markers or signs of active disease, and this finding impacts the quality of life of patients with even quiescent IBD.[62,63] This am-biguity in the immediate cause of ongoing abdominal complaints, whether caused by inflammation or visceral hypersensitivity, poses a challenge to treating physicians, as the patients' symptoms may not necessarily be due to active CD but rather due to IBS. Interestingly, Keohane and colleagues,[64] found that almost 60% of a subgroup of pa-tients with CD in clinical remission and with a low C-reactive protein (CRP) meet the ROME II criteria for IBS. This finding is similar to the visceral hypersensitivity seen in patients with IBS, especially in the postinfectious subtype, in which an inflammatory trigger leads to a both peripheral and central sensitization manifesting as the symp-toms of diarrhea and abdominal pain IBS.[65] Given the prevalence of IBS as high as 10% to 15% of the general US population, then if by chance alone, there is a high probability that some patients with IBD will also have IBS.[66] Moreover, many patients who are diagnosed with IBD, may have been initially misdiagnosed as IBS several years prior due to the overlap in symptomatology or as a prodromal period in CD.[67] Oftentimes, aggressive treatment of the underlying inflammation suspected in patients with IBD despite lack of serologic, endoscopic or imaging diagnosis, is a mainstay of management. Many scientists propose that IBS-D maybe an "incomplete" CD.[68] Although, some clinicians may choose to treat the overlapping symptoms of IBD and IBS empirically, the response to treatment may not necessarily be indicative of active disease but based on a recent meta-analysis, may be secondary to a placebo effect, which can be as high as 33% in IBS trials (155 trials), 35% in UC trials (82 trials), and 25% in CD.[69,70]

Diagnosis and Differentiation from Inflammatory Bowel Disease and Small Intestinal Bacterial Overgrowth

Treatment of quiescent IBD by increasing the dose of immunosuppressive agents will likely increase the risk for side effects, including malignancy, infections, and malabsorption. Therefore, how do we identify those patients who present with symptoms due to an FBD versus those with active inflammation or long-term consequences of their IBD? A few recent developments in new biomarkers for the treatment of patients with IBS-D have enhanced our ability to differentiate IBS from non-IBS, IBD. This development of validated biomarkers that can help identify and separate those patients with FBD from those with active inflammation is at its preliminary stages but would be invaluable for clinical care, as it is incorporated into the new ROME IV criteria.[61] Some of these are existing biomarkers, CRP level in serum and fecal calprotectin, which are associated with objective mucosal inflammation in patients with IBD and may have high sensitivity and specificity as a screening tool for IBD in adults and children.[71] These tests could even differentiate IBS-D from microscopic colitis, thus avoiding need for endoscopy in a subset of patients.[72] Other newly developed markers are antibodies against cytolethal distending toxin B, which is produced by all gram-negative bacteria with subsequent development of other antibodies, through a molecular mimicry, to vinculin.[73] Vinculin is a cytoskeletal protein that binds adhesion molecules to actin, thereby supporting the intestinal barrier against injury. High levels of both antibodies have been detected in patients with IBS-D subtype but not in IBD, with a specificity of 92% and a sensitivity of 44%. Although the test does not differentiate celiac disease from IBS, it may be a reliable test for "ruling in" IBS, therefore minimizing use of invasive testing as would be necessary for ruling out IBD. Correct identification of IBS would have huge implications for the treatment and identification of quiescent CD, which would mimic IBS.

Another possibly distinct (but not mutually exclusive) entity coexisting with IBD and IBS may be small intestinal bacterial overgrowth (SIBO) defined as clinical or laboratory evidence of malabsorption due to an increased population of small bowel bacteria. The clinical presentation of a patient with SIBO can be similar to IBS, IBD, celiac disease, carbohydrate malabsorption, and even partial mechanical obstruction. These symptoms include abdominal fullness, bloating, upper periumbilical or epigastric abdominal pain, diarrhea, weight loss, and/or nausea with vomiting and weight loss.[74] The presence of bacteria in the small bowel results in intestinal fermentation with production of gases, production of metabolites in addition to degradation of carbohydrates, production of short-chain fatty acids altering motility and leading to symptoms in IBS (4%–54%), and possibly UC (15%) and CD (28%).[75–77] These rates depend on the method of diagnosis used: breath testing or duodenal/jejunal aspirates and cultures. IBD itself is a risk factor for having a positive = jejunal aspirate. This "gold standard" is both invasive and costly with limitations depending on type of method for cultures obtained.[78] Hydrogen breath testing by both lactulose and glucose breath testing methods is an alternative to obtaining aspirates in patients with suspected SIBO and rely on high levels of methane and hydrogen. However, both lactulose (an osmotic laxative) and glucose have been shown to accelerate intestinal transit and especially in patients with diarrhea (IBD or IBS) could result in false-positive findings due to rapid arrival of substrate to the right colon.[79] We do not advocate breath testing in patients with symptoms of diarrhea and known IBD. A recent North American Consensus Meeting has made an effort to standardize testing for SIBO, noting jejunal cultures of $\geq 10^3$ coliforms/mL colonic bacteria and not $\geq 10^5$ as the new standard SIBO definition with further standardizing of breath testing.[80]

Our Recommendations

Given the complexity and overlap of IBS, IBD, and SIBO, we first advocate dietary measures with 2 diets found to be most effective in patients with IBD and IBS: Low FODMAP diet and less consistently, a gluten-free diet[81] (**Fig. 4**). Two probiotics

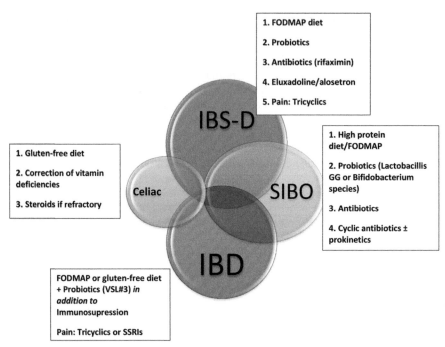

Fig. 4. Management of overlapping diseases.

most studied in patients with IBD and IBS, *Bifidobacterium infantis* and the combination probiotic VSL#3, are advocated as first-line treatments; however, one should note that probiotics treat only pain and bloating but not fecal urgency or frequency.[82] These therapies may be followed by treatments for concomitant IBS-D targeting serotonin (alosetron), opiate agonists (eluxadoline), and nonsystemically absorbed antibiotics (rifaximin), which are now the 3 FDA-approved treatments for IBS-D. Incorporating use of antidepressants, such as the TCAs especially in patients with IBD with frequent comorbidities, such as anxiety and depression, also may be helpful to treat the visceral hypersensitivity, and as tricyclics are less likely to cause more diarrhea.[56] In patients found to have significant weight loss with suspected small bowel dysmotility causing SIBO, or in those with normal transit and imaging excluding a stricture as the cause of continued symptoms, empiric treatment of SIBO with a nonsystemic antibiotic such as rifaximin versus other antibiotics should be started, although trials of rifaximin in exclusively patients with SIBO do not exist in well-designed studies.[83] If the patient continues to decline, however, without evidence of an inflammatory cause, jejunal aspirates should be done with cultures added for possible fungal overgrowth. Checking for micronutrient deficiencies is also important, as patients with SIBO often have high or normal folate and vitamin K levels, as they are produced by bacteria.

EVALUATION OF ANORECTAL DISEASES IN INFLAMMATORY BOWEL DISEASE

The anorectum is commonly involved in patients with UC (100%) and CD (15%–80%), where inflammation, fistulous disease, or surgery in the anorectal area leads to fibrosis, rectal hypersensitivity, and a noncompliant rectum.[84] Although advances in the treatment of IBD with use of biologic agents, and surgical reconstructive techniques, such as IPAA have modified the treatment of fistulas and other anorectal diseases in patients with IBD, still, fecal incontinence, defecatory dysfunction such as puborectalis muscle dysfunction, and pelvic pain occur commonly in IBD and greatly impact a patient's quality of life.[85,86]

Fecal Incontinence in Inflammatory Bowel Disease

Fecal incontinence is one of the main anorectal complaints of patients with IBD and is reported in up to 25%, higher than the average population.[87] Besides diarrhea itself, which may be multifactorial and due to ongoing inflammation, pouchitis, bile acid malabsorption, concomitant FBD, lactose intolerance, and SIBO, sphincter damage due to presence of fistula and anal fibrosis can also contribute. Earlier reports based on anorectal manometry testing have found patients with UC and active disease have increased rectal hypersensitivity and contractility whereas rectal compliance is impaired in those with both quiescent and active UC suggesting chronic changes of rectal wall with fibrosis may be responsible.[88] Patients with active disease and anorectal manometry showing lower rectal compliance have a higher risk of incontinence, similar to those with higher fatigue of sphincter muscles with or without sphincter defects seen on ultrasonography.[89]

In patients with UC status-post IPAA, fecal incontinence and functional outcomes are not different according to a meta-analysis of 53 studies with a durability of 90% if done in the experienced setting.[90] Furthermore, fecal incontinence is not seen more frequently in patients with IPAA with a hand sewn versus stapled anastomoses.[90,91] In patients with suspected sphincter damage either due to obstetric surgery or other structural defects found by manometry or ultrasonography of anorectum, a modified IPAA has been suggested by some can be done to improve risk of incontinence.[92] Therefore, diagnostic testing preoperatively with anorectal manometry can be useful in ruling out sphincter defects before IPAA, especially if sphincter defects are suspected[93] (**Fig. 5**). Few long-term follow-ups of patients with IBD and fecal

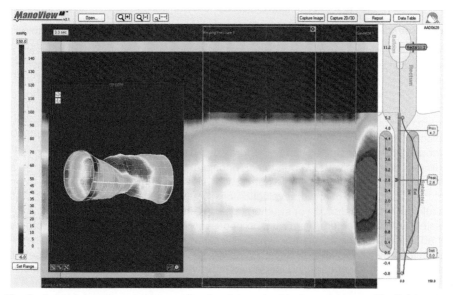

Fig. 5. Anorectal manometry image showing internal sphincter weakness with slight anterior and posterior defect on 3-dimensional imaging in a patient with CD with severe perianal disease status-post ileostomy. Manometry was done for symptoms of fecal incontinence and before ileostomy takedown.

incontinence have been performed, with one study showing that after 14 years, 54% of patients with IBD with perianal lesions continue to have mild complaints.[94] Most of these patients, 39%, had prior history of fistulous disease at baseline. Depression and even suicidal symptoms are higher in patients with CD and perianal disease, therefore many advocate use of a validated fecal continence questionnaire in patients with IBD (ICIQ-IBD).[95,96]

Our Recommendations

Several therapies are available for treatment of fecal incontinence, including biofeed-back therapy, fiber supplementation for bulking, and loperamide. Other minimally invasive techniques for treatment of fecal incontinence have been studied in IBD in small case series including sacral nerve stimulation, posterior tibial nerve stimulation, or bulking agents, showing some efficacy in a subset of patients with IPAA.[97,98]

Pelvic Floor Disorders in Inflammatory Bowel Disease

Pelvic floor disorders, such as dyssynergia, causing an obstructive defecation and subsequent fecal impaction with overflow diarrhea are also common among patients with IBD, although the true prevalence of these disorders is unknown.[99] One study of a group of patients with IBD with quiescent disease (23 CD, 6 UC) found defecatory disorders by manometry testing to be 67%, 10%, and 6%, respectively, in those with constipation, stool frequency, and incontinence with and without rectal pain. All but one met criteria for dyssynergia with inability to expel the balloon during defecation and with anismus during push maneuvers. Abdominal radiograph showed that most patients in this study with complaints of frequent stooling had overflow diarrhea due to constipation. The authors stress the importance of a good physical examination, including a rectal examination, in the evaluation of patients with all anorectal diseases to rule out anorectal cancers found more frequently in patients with IBD, ruling out prolapse of rectum or pouch, and other structural or functional anorectal diseases.

Our Recommendations

Treatment of patients with these disorders, however, should begin with conservative therapy of increase of fiber and fluid intake and osmotic laxatives as tolerated. If symptoms persist, physiologic testing with anorectal manometry and balloon expulsion to evaluate for pelvic floor disorders should be performed. Biofeedback therapy should be initiated in most cases perhaps even before use of laxatives, as it is longer lasting and may completely resolve the defecatory symptoms.[100] Transit studies are rarely indicated for patients with CD or UC to evaluate for slow-transit constipation, and although Sitzmarker studies can be performed, the wireless motility capsule is contraindicated in patients with CD due to risk of capsule retention, although this may be a better tool for evaluation of whole gut motility. Use of MRI defecography is yet to be determined but may help with evaluation of rectal volume and dispensability as well as rule out fistulous disease or structural defects. In patients with pelvic pain, a multidisciplinary management team may be necessary to avoid unnecessary laparotomy for adhesions in patients already at high risk of wound healing and infection. Rehabilitation therapy with specialists trained in pelvic pain with avoidance of narcotic use will greatly impact patient care and lead to an improved quality of life for these patients.

SUMMARY

Patients with IBD have overlapping symptoms with both motility and functional bowel diseases. In patients with quiescent disease or continued symptoms despite dose escalation, diagnostic testing and a thorough evaluation for other concomitant gastrointestinal disorders should be performed to further improve management of these patients with chronic illnesses and to minimize the risk of further unnecessary immunosuppression or that of empiric treatments that may predispose patients to infections or further malnutrition.

REFERENCES

1. Bryant RV, van Langenberg DR, Holtmann GJ, et al. Functional gastrointestinal disorders in inflammatory bowel disease: impact on quality of life and psychological status. J Gastroenterol Hepatol 2011;26(5):916–23.
2. Barratt SM, Leeds JS, Robinson K, et al. Reflux and irritable bowel syndrome are negative predictors of quality of life in coeliac disease and inflammatory bowel disease. Eur J Gastroenterol Hepatol 2011;23(2):159–65.
3. El-Serag HB, Sweet S, Winchester CC, et al. Update on the epidemiology of gastro-oesophageal reflux disease: a systematic review. Gut 2014;63(6): 871–80.
4. Davis KG. Crohn's disease of the foregut. Surg Clin North Am 2015;95(6): 1183–93, vi.
5. De Felice KM, Katzka DA, Raffals LE. Crohn's disease of the esophagus: clinical features and treatment outcomes in the biologic era. Inflamm Bowel Dis 2015; 21(9):2106–13.
6. Decker GA, Loftus EV Jr, Pasha TM, et al. Crohn's disease of the esophagus: clinical features and outcomes. Inflamm Bowel Dis 2001;7(2):113–9.
7. Ramaswamy K, Jacobson K, Jevon G, et al. Esophageal Crohn disease in children: a clinical spectrum. J Pediatr Gastroenterol Nutr 2003;36(4):454–8.
8. Lenaerts C, Roy CC, Vaillancourt M, et al. High incidence of upper gastrointestinal tract involvement in children with Crohn disease. Pediatrics 1989;83(5): 777–81.
9. Sawczenko A, Sandhu BK. Presenting features of inflammatory bowel disease in Great Britain and Ireland. Arch Dis Child 2003;88(11):995–1000.
10. Korelitz BI, Waye JD, Kreuning J, et al. Crohn's disease in endoscopic biopsies of the gastric antrum and duodenum. Am J Gastroenterol 1981;76(2):103–9.
11. Cameron DJ. Upper and lower gastrointestinal endoscopy in children and adolescents with Crohn's disease: a prospective study. J Gastroenterol Hepatol 1991;6(4):355–8.
12. Turner D, Griffiths AM. Esophageal, gastric, and duodenal manifestations of IBD and the role of upper endoscopy in IBD diagnosis. Curr Gastroenterol Rep 2009;11(3):234–7.
13. Gasche C, Scholmerich J, Brynskov J, et al. A simple classification of Crohn's disease: report of the Working Party for the World Congresses of Gastroenterology, Vienna 1998. Inflamm Bowel Dis 2000;6(1):8–15.
14. Silverberg MS, Satsangi J, Ahmad T, et al. Toward an integrated clinical, molecular and serological classification of inflammatory bowel disease: report of a Working Party of the 2005 Montreal World Congress of Gastroenterology. Can J Gastroenterol 2005;19(Suppl A):5A–36A.
15. Makuuchi H, Shimada H, Chino O, et al. Endoscopic classification of reflux esophagitis and its new developments. Nihon Geka Gakkai Zasshi 1997; 98(11):926–31 [in Japanese].
16. Takubo K, Honma N, Aryal G, et al. Is there a set of histologic changes that are invariably reflux associated? Arch Pathol Lab Med 2005;129(2):159–63.

17. Geboes K, Janssens J, Rutgeerts P, et al. Crohn's disease of the esophagus. J Clin Gastroenterol 1986;8(1):31–7.

18. Poritz LS, Sehgal R, Berg AS, et al. Chronic use of PPI and H2 antagonists decreases the risk of pouchitis after IPAA for ulcerative colitis. J Gastrointest Surg 2013;17(6):1027–31.

19. Miehsler W, Puspok A, Oberhuber T, et al. Impact of different therapeutic regimens on the outcome of patients with Crohn's disease of the upper gastrointestinal tract. Inflamm Bowel Dis 2001;7(2):99–105.

20. Mottet C, Juillerat P, Pittet V, et al. Upper gastrointestinal Crohn's disease. Digestion 2007;76(2):136–40.

21. Sheen E, Triadafilopoulos G. Adverse effects of long-term proton pump inhibitor therapy. Dig Dis Sci 2011;56(4):931–50.

22. Wyatt CM. Proton pump inhibitors and chronic kidney disease: is it time to sound the alarm? Kidney Int 2016;89(4):732–3.

23. Targownik LE, Bernstein CN, Leslie WD. Inflammatory bowel disease and the risk of osteoporosis and fracture. Maturitas 2013;76(4):315–9.

24. Trifan A, Stanciu C, Stoica O, et al. Impact of *Clostridium difficile* infection on inflammatory bowel disease outcome: a review. World J Gastroenterol 2014; 20(33):11736–42.

25. Linsky A, Gupta K, Lawler EV, et al. Proton pump inhibitors and risk for recurrent *Clostridium difficile* infection. Arch Intern Med 2010;170(9):772–8.

26. Lombardo L, Foti M, Ruggia O, et al. Increased incidence of small intestinal bacterial overgrowth during proton pump inhibitor therapy. Clin Gastroenterol Hepatol 2010;8(6):504–8.

27. Aziz Q, Fass R, Gyawali CP, et al. Functional esophageal disorders. Gastroenterology 2016. [Epub ahead of print].

28. Diaz L, Hernandez-Oquet RE, Deshpande AR, et al. Upper gastrointestinal involvement in Crohn disease: histopathologic and endoscopic findings. South Med J 2015;108(11):695–700.

29. Annunziata ML, Caviglia R, Papparella LG, et al. Upper gastrointestinal involvement of Crohn's disease: a prospective study on the role of upper endoscopy in the diagnostic work-up. Dig Dis Sci 2012;57(6):1618–23.

30. Camilleri M, Parkman HP, Shafi MA, et al. Clinical guideline: management of gastroparesis. Am J Gastroenterol 2013;108(1):18–37 [quiz: 8].

31. Gryboski JD, Burger J, McCallum R, et al. Gastric emptying in childhood inflammatory bowel disease: nutritional and pathologic correlates. Am J Gastroenterol 1992;87(9):1148–53.

32. Keller J, Beglinger C, Holst JJ, et al. Mechanisms of gastric emptying disturbances in chronic and acute inflammation of the distal gastrointestinal tract. Am J Physiol Gastrointest Liver Physiol 2009;297(5):G861–8.

33. De Schepper HU, De Man JG, Van Nassauw L, et al. Acute distal colitis impairs gastric emptying in rats via an extrinsic neuronal reflex pathway involving the pelvic nerve. Gut 2007;56(2):195–202.

34. Porcher C, Baldo M, Henry M, et al. Deficiency of interstitial cells of Cajal in the small intestine of patients with Crohn's disease. Am J Gastroenterol 2002;97(1): 118–25.

35. Grill BB, Lange R, Markowitz R, et al. Delayed gastric emptying in children with Crohn's disease. J Clin Gastroenterol 1985;7(3):216–26.

36. Keller J, Binnewies U, Rosch M, et al. Gastric emptying and disease activity in inflammatory bowel disease. Eur J Clin Invest 2015;45(12):1234–42.

37. Tomita R, Fujisaki S, Tanjoh K. Gastric emptying function after ileal J pouch-anal anastomosis for ulcerative colitis. Surgery 2004;135(1):81–6.
38. Tougas G, Eaker EY, Abell TL, et al. Assessment of gastric emptying using a low fat meal: establishment of international control values. Am J Gastroenterol 2000; 95(6):1456–62.
39. Saad RJ, Hasler WL. A technical review and clinical assessment of the wireless motility capsule. Gastroenterol Hepatol (N Y) 2011;7(12):795–804.
40. Wytiaz V, Homko C, Duffy F, et al. Foods provoking and alleviating symptoms in gastroparesis: patient experiences. Dig Dis Sci 2015;60(4):1052–8.
41. Parkman HP, Van Natta ML, Abell TL, et al. Effect of nortriptyline on symptoms of idiopathic gastroparesis: the NORIG randomized clinical trial. JAMA 2013; 310(24):2640–9.
42. Sturm A, Holtmann G, Goebell H, et al. Prokinetics in patients with gastroparesis: a systematic analysis. Digestion 1999;60(5):422–7.
43. Ray WA, Murray KT, Hall K, et al. Azithromycin and the risk of cardiovascular death. N Engl J Med 2012;366(20):1881–90.
44. Brown KA, Khanafer N, Daneman N, et al. Meta-analysis of antibiotics and the risk of community-associated *Clostridium difficile* infection. Antimicrob Agents Chemother 2013;57(5):2326–32.
45. Rao AS, Camilleri M. Review article: metoclopramide and tardive dyskinesia. Aliment Pharmacol Ther 2010;31(1):11–9.
46. Silvers D, Kipnes M, Broadstone V, et al. Domperidone in the management of symptoms of diabetic gastroparesis: efficacy, tolerability, and quality-of-life outcomes in a multicenter controlled trial. DOM-USA-5 Study Group. Clin Ther 1998;20(3):438–53.
47. Waseem S, Moshiree B, Draganov PV. Gastroparesis: current diagnostic challenges and management considerations. World J Gastroenterol 2009;15(1): 25–37.
48. McCallum RW, Fink SM, Lerner E, et al. Effects of metoclopramide and bethanechol on delayed gastric emptying present in gastroesophageal reflux patients. Gastroenterology 1983;84(6):1573–7.
49. Camilleri M. Novel diet, drugs, and gastric interventions for gastroparesis. Clin Gastroenterol Hepatol 2016. [Epub ahead of print].
50. Lembo A, Camilleri M, McCallum R, et al. Relamorelin reduces vomiting frequency and severity and accelerates gastric emptying in adults with diabetic gastroparesis. Gastroenterology 2016;151(1):87–96.e6.
51. Xue L, Locke GR, Camilleri M, et al. Effect of modulation of serotonergic, cholinergic, and nitrergic pathways on murine fundic size and compliance measured by ultrasonomicrometry. Am J Physiol Gastrointest Liver Physiol 2006;290(1): G74–82.
52. Saad RJ, Chey WD. Review article: current and emerging therapies for functional dyspepsia. Aliment Pharmacol Ther 2006;24(3):475–92.
53. Stanghellini V, Chan FKL, Hasler WL, et al. Gastroduodenal disorders. Gastroenterology 2016;150(6):1380–92.
54. Talley NJ, Ford AC. Functional dyspepsia. N Engl J Med 2015;373(19):1853–63.
55. Mak AD, Wu JC, Chan Y, et al. Dyspepsia is strongly associated with major depression and generalised anxiety disorder—a community study. Aliment Pharmacol Ther 2012;36(8):800–10.
56. Panara AJ, Yarur AJ, Rieders B, et al. The incidence and risk factors for developing depression after being diagnosed with inflammatory bowel disease: a cohort study. Aliment Pharmacol Ther 2014;39(8):802–10.

57. Talley NJ, Locke GR, Saito YA, et al. Effect of amitriptyline and escitalopram on functional dyspepsia: a multicenter, randomized controlled study. Gastroenterology 2015;149(2):340–9.e2.

58. Melzer J, Rosch W, Reichling J, et al. Meta-analysis: phytotherapy of functional dyspepsia with the herbal drug preparation STW 5 (Iberogast). Aliment Pharmacol Ther 2004;20(11–12):1279–87.

59. Rodriguez L, Diaz J, Nurko S. Safety and efficacy of cyproheptadine for treating dyspeptic symptoms in children. J Pediatr 2013;163(1):261–7.

60. Tack J, Janssen P, Masaoka T, et al. Efficacy of buspirone, a fundus-relaxing drug, in patients with functional dyspepsia. Clin Gastroenterol Hepatol 2012; 10(11):1239–45.

61. Mearin F, Lacy BE, Chang L, et al. Bowel disorders. Gastroenterology 2016. [Epub ahead of print].

62. Piche T, Ducrotte P, Sabate JM, et al. Impact of functional bowel symptoms on quality of life and fatigue in quiescent Crohn disease and irritable bowel syndrome. Neurogastroenterol Motil 2010;22(6):626–e174.

63. Halpin SJ, Ford AC. Prevalence of symptoms meeting criteria for irritable bowel syndrome in inflammatory bowel disease: systematic review and meta-analysis. Am J Gastroenterol 2012;107(10):1474–82.

64. Keohane J, O'Mahony C, O'Mahony L, et al. Irritable bowel syndrome-type symptoms in patients with inflammatory bowel disease: a real association or reflection of occult inflammation? Am J Gastroenterol 2010;105(8):1788, 1789–94; [quiz: 95].

65. Price DD, Zhou Q, Moshiree B, et al. Peripheral and central contributions to hyperalgesia in irritable bowel syndrome. J Pain 2006;7(8):529–35.

66. Hungin AP, Chang L, Locke GR, et al. Irritable bowel syndrome in the United States: prevalence, symptom patterns and impact. Aliment Pharmacol Ther 2005;21(11):1365–75.

67. Pimentel M, Chang M, Chow EJ, et al. Identification of a prodromal period in Crohn's disease but not ulcerative colitis. Am J Gastroenterol 2000;95(12): 3458–62.

68. Olbe L. Concept of Crohn's disease being conditioned by four main components, and irritable bowel syndrome being an incomplete Crohn's disease. Scand J Gastroenterol 2008;43(2):234–41.

69. Talley NJ, Abreu MT, Achkar JP, et al. An evidence-based systematic review on medical therapies for inflammatory bowel disease. Am J Gastroenterol 2011; 106(Suppl 1):S2–25 [quiz: S6].

70. Bielefeldt K, Dudekula A, Levinthal DJ. 364 power of placebo: a meta-analysis of trials in irritable bowel syndrome and ulcerative colitis. Gastroenterology 2016; 150(4):S81.

71. van Rheenen PF, Van de Vijver E, Fidler V. Faecal calprotectin for screening of patients with suspected inflammatory bowel disease: diagnostic meta-analysis. BMJ 2010;341:c3369.

72. von Arnim U, Wex T, Ganzert C, et al. Fecal calprotectin: a marker for clinical differentiation of microscopic colitis and irritable bowel syndrome. Clin Exp Gastroenterol 2016;9:97–103.

73. Pimentel M, Morales W, Rezaie A, et al. Development and validation of a biomarker for diarrhea-predominant irritable bowel syndrome in human subjects. PLoS One 2015;10(5):e0126438.

74. Moshiree B, Ringel Y. Small bowel bacterial overgrowth syndrome. In: Rao SSC, Parkman H, McCallum R, editors. Handbook of gastrointestinal motility and functional disorders. Thorofare, NJ: Slack Incorporated; 2015. p. 187–200.

75. Ford AC, Spiegel BM, Talley NJ, et al. Small intestinal bacterial overgrowth in irritable bowel syndrome: systematic review and meta-analysis. Clin Gastroenterol Hepatol 2009;7(12):1279–86.

76. Rana SV, Sharma S, Kaur J, et al. Relationship of cytokines, oxidative stress and GI motility with bacterial overgrowth in ulcerative colitis patients. J Crohns Colitis 2014;8(8):859–65.

77. Klaus J, Spaniol U, Adler G, et al. Small intestinal bacterial overgrowth mimicking acute flare as a pitfall in patients with Crohn's Disease. BMC Gastroenterol 2009;9:61.

78. Choung RS, Ruff KC, Malhotra A, et al. Clinical predictors of small intestinal bacterial overgrowth by duodenal aspirate culture. Aliment Pharmacol Ther 2011; 33(9):1059–67.

79. Lin EC, Massey BT. Scintigraphy demonstrates high rate of false-positive results from glucose breath tests for small bowel bacterial overgrowth. Clin Gastroenterol Hepatol 2016;14(2):203–8.

80. Rezaie A, Buresi M, Lembo A, et al. 450 Hydrogen- and methane-based breath testing (BT) in gastrointestinal (GI) disorders: report of the North American Consensus Meeting. Gastroenterology 2016;150(4):S97.

81. Knight-Sepulveda K, Kais S, Santaolalla R, et al. Diet and inflammatory bowel disease. Gastroenterol Hepatol (N Y) 2015;11(8):511–20.

82. Floch MH, Walker WA, Sanders ME, et al. Recommendations for probiotic use–2015 update: proceedings and consensus opinion. J Clin Gastroenterol 2015; 49(Suppl 1):S69–73.

83. Shah SC, Day LW, Somsouk M, et al. Meta-analysis: antibiotic therapy for small intestinal bacterial overgrowth. Aliment Pharmacol Ther 2013;38(8):925–34.

84. Sandborn WJ, Fazio VW, Feagan BG, et al. AGA technical review on perianal Crohn's disease. Gastroenterology 2003;125(5):1508–30.

85. Norton C, Dibley LB, Bassett P. Faecal incontinence in inflammatory bowel disease: associations and effect on quality of life. J Crohns Colitis 2013;7(8): e302–11.

86. Bondurri A, Maffioli A, Danelli P. Pelvic floor dysfunction in inflammatory bowel disease. Minerva Gastroenterol Dietol 2015;61(4):249–59.

87. Singh B, Mc CMNJ, Jewell DP, et al. Perianal Crohn's disease. Br J Surg 2004; 91(7):801–14.

88. Loening-Baucke V, Metcalf AM, Shirazi S. Anorectal manometry in active and quiescent ulcerative colitis. Am J Gastroenterol 1989;84(8):892–7.

89. Papathanasopoulos A, Van Oudenhove L, Katsanos K, et al. Severity of fecal urgency and incontinence in inflammatory bowel disease: clinical, manometric and sonographic predictors. Inflamm Bowel Dis 2013;19(11):2450–6.

90. de Zeeuw S, Ahmed Ali U, Donders RA, et al. Update of complications and functional outcome of the ileo-pouch anal anastomosis: overview of evidence and meta-analysis of 96 observational studies. Int J Colorectal Dis 2012;27(7): 843–53.

91. Shawki S, Belizon A, Person B, et al. What are the outcomes of reoperative restorative proctocolectomy and ileal pouch-anal anastomosis surgery? Dis Colon Rectum 2009;52(5):884–90.

92. Kobakov G, Kostov D, Temelkov T. Manometric study in ulcerative colitis patients with modified ileal pouch–anal anastomosis. Int J Colorectal Dis 2006; 21(8):767–73.

93. Silvis R, van Eekelen JW, Delemarre JB, et al. Endosonography of the anal sphincter after ileal pouch-anal anastomosis. Relation with anal manometry and fecal continence. Dis Colon Rectum 1995;38(4):383–8.

94. Lam TJ, van Bodegraven AA, Felt-Bersma RJ. Anorectal complications and function in patients suffering from inflammatory bowel disease: a series of patients with long-term follow-up. Int J Colorectal Dis 2014;29(8):923–9.

95. Mahadev S, Young JM, Selby W, et al. Self-reported depressive symptoms and suicidal feelings in perianal Crohn's disease. Colorectal Dis 2012;14(3):331–5.

96. Dibley L, Norton C, Cotterill N, et al. Development and initial validation of a disease-specific bowel continence questionnaire for inflammatory bowel disease patients: the ICIQ-IBD. Eur J Gastroenterol Hepatol 2016;28(2):233–9.

97. Vitton V, Damon H, Roman S, et al. Transcutaneous posterior tibial nerve stimulation for fecal incontinence in inflammatory bowel disease patients: a therapeutic option? Inflamm Bowel Dis 2009;15(3):402–5.

98. Lebas A, Rogosnitzky M, Chater C, et al. Efficacy of sacral nerve stimulation for poor functional results of J-pouch ileoanal anastomosis. Tech Coloproctol 2014; 18(4):355–60.

99. Perera LP, Ananthakrishnan AN, Guilday C, et al. Dyssynergic defecation: a treatable cause of persistent symptoms when inflammatory bowel disease is in remission. Dig Dis Sci 2013;58(12):3600–5.

100. Chiarioni G, Whitehead WE, Pezza V, et al. Biofeedback is superior to laxatives for normal transit constipation due to pelvic floor dyssynergia. Gastroenterology 2006;130(3):657–64.

Dilation of Strictures in Patients with Inflammatory Bowel Disease
Who, When and How

Nayantara Coelho-Prabhu, MBBS, John A. Martin, MD*

KEYWORDS

- Strictures • Anastomoses • Biliary strictures • Dilation • Needle knife

KEY POINTS

- Strictures—de novo versus anastomotic, locations, inflammatory versus fibrotic—in inflammatory bowel disease (IBD) are discussed.
- The pros and cons of dilation, symptoms, confirmation of inflammation with cross-sectional imaging, and j pouch and anal-pouch strictures are discussed.
- The technical details, size of balloons, use of fluoroscopy of dilation are presented.
- Other adjuncts procedures include steroids, needle knife, and stent.
- About 10% to 15% patients with IBD develop primary sclerosing cholangitis, which results in stricture formation in the biliary tree.

INTRODUCTION

Patients with Crohn's disease may develop strictures either before surgery or after surgery. We will discuss when and how to dilate strictures in IBD patients. We will discuss endoscopic retrograde cholangiopancreatography (ERCP) in patients with primary sclerosing cholangitis (PSC) and the proper evaluation and management of strictures in this condition.

Transmural inflammation is a hallmark of Crohn's disease, which leads to stricturing of the bowel wall. These strictures may be inflammatory, fibrotic, or, most often, a combination of both. In patients with Crohn's disease, around one-third will develop strictures within 10 years of diagnosis.[1] These strictures occur most commonly at the colon, ileocolonic region, and ileum[2] and are termed de novo strictures. Also, the cumulative risk of surgery for bowel resection within 10 years of diagnosis is

Division of Gastroenterology and Hepatology, Mayo Clinic, 200 First Street Southwest, Rochester, MN 55905, USA
* Corresponding author.
E-mail address: martin.john3@mayo.edu

Gastrointest Endoscopy Clin N Am 26 (2016) 739–759
http://dx.doi.org/10.1016/j.giec.2016.06.011
1052-5157/16/© 2016 Elsevier Inc. All rights reserved.

around 50%.[3] In these patients, recurrence of disease occurs in 44% to 55%, which is often associated with restenosis at the anastomotic site. At times, anastomotic strictures can occur owing to altered blood supply at the level of the anastomosis, and these are usually not associated with active inflammation.

In ulcerative colitis, rates of colectomy in more recent cohorts in the era of biologics is around 10% to 16.6%.[4–7] Among these patients, anastomotic strictures can form at the pouch–anal anastomosis and rarely at the pouch–inlet anastomosis. In about 5% to 10% of colitis, indeterminate colitis is diagnosed. Both classic ulcerative colitis patients and indeterminate colitis patients can progress to Crohn's disease of the ileal–pouch–anal anastomosis, often manifesting with strictures in the pouch and prepouch ileum.

Strictures in IBD occur as a result of scarring and fibrosis in the setting of chronic inflammation in the bowel wall. As a result, most strictures demonstrate a combination of fibrosis and active inflammation. Endoscopically, active ongoing inflammation is manifest as ulcerations and edema at the narrowed site. Radiographically, too, active inflammation can be demonstrated in a strictured segment both on computed tomography enterography and MR enterography. In a lesser number of situations, the stricture is almost completely fibrotic without any evidence of active inflammation. The presence of active inflammation endoscopically is an important factor in dilation of these strictures because it can limit the extent of dilation that is performed. Actively inflamed bowel wall is more friable and more likely to result in a complication of perforation.

Strictures in IBD patients have diverse manifestations. When they affect the gastric outlet or duodenum, patients can present with symptoms of gastric outlet obstruction including nausea, vomiting, and an inability to eat. When they affect the small bowel, patients usually present with intermittent partial small bowel obstruction symptoms including abdominal pain, abdominal distention, obstipation, and vomiting. At times, the symptoms may be more subtle, with just postprandial abdominal cramping, especially a few hours after intake of high residue foods. Colonic strictures are the most well-tolerated, and hence often present very late. Patients complain of change in the caliber or stool, and at times increasing constipation. When the stricture is at the pouch–anal anastomosis, tenesmus, and a feeling of incomplete evacuation are common symptoms. Also, excessive straining and urgency with watery stool can occur in this scenario.

Imaging of the strictures is very important before attempting endoscopic therapy. This is both to delineate the location, extent, and possibly diameter of the stricture, and also to document the presence and extent of concurrent inflammation. Ideal imaging is cross-sectional in the form of a computed tomography enterography or MR enterography.[8] Both of these techniques are able to provide a fairly precise location of the stricture, and an assessment of degree of inflammation. Small bowel series have been used in the past, but cannot provide any information on inflammation within the bowel wall. Barium enemas can be useful in colonic and pouch strictures because the sensitivity of computed tomography and MR is lower. They can outline the length and location of strictures well, and should be considered before therapy if this information is unknown. Imaging, both cross-sectional and contrast radiography, can also help to identify other complications of IBD including fistulae, abscesses, or sinus tracts, which can occur in conjunction with stricturing disease.

When to Dilate

Strictures in IBD should be treated if they are symptomatic, as described. If active inflammation is present, medical therapy should be optimized first. In the case of anastomotic strictures, even if the patients are not overtly symptomatic, endoscopic dilation should be performed if the endoscope is unable to pass through the stricture, to allow for examination of the more proximal bowel and to prevent symptoms from developing down the road.

How to Dilate

The first principle in endoscopic dilation is choosing the correct endoscope to reach the site of the stricture. Upper endoscopes are used for gastric and proximal duodenal strictures. For distal jejunal and proximal jejunal strictures, a push enteroscopy using the pediatric colonoscope is usually necessary. Often times, however, in these patients, the bowel can be fairly angulated, and we recommend using the more flexible enteroscope (either with single- or double-balloon technology) to reach these sites. In the colon and for ileocolonic anastomotic strictures, the pediatric colonoscope is usually the best choice given its flexibility. Here too, if the ileocolonic anastomosis is a side-to-side anastomosis and fairly angulated, use of an enteroscope may facilitate access to and passage through this site. Ileal strictures almost always require an enteroscope to reach the site. Strictures in the left colon can often be sharply angulated especially in the sigmoid colon or at colorectal anastomoses. Here, the more flexible upper endoscope is favorable.

Dilation is performed using graduated, through-the-scope balloon dilators, except at the anal verge, which is discussed elsewhere in this paper. If the exact diameter of the stricture is unknown beforehand, it is advisable to use a suite with fluoroscopic capability that can be used if necessary. Once the stricture is identified, if the endoscope is able to traverse it, the balloon can be advanced beyond the stricture, and then pulled back to straddle the stricture before inflation. If the stricture cannot be traversed with the scope, then the balloon should be advanced across the stricture. This is safely done if there is minimal surrounding inflammation and no resistance to balloon passage is encountered. If the stricture seems to be long or if any resistance is encountered, then the dilation should be undertaken over a guidewire. The guidewire can be passed through the stricture under fluoroscopic guidance to ensure the presence of the wire in the bowel lumen past the stricture. Over the guidewire, the balloon can then be advanced across the stricture.

The choice of the diameter of the balloon depends on the initial diameter of the stricture, the presence or absence of ulcers and inflammation, and the previous maximal diameter achieved if this is a repeat dilation. The diameter of the stricture can be estimated based on the diameter of the endoscope being used as these diameters are readily available. Another trick is to use the diameter of a known device such as an open biopsy cable as a reference to guess the approximate stricture diameter. The initial balloon diameter chosen should be a little larger than the estimated baseline diameter of the stricture. The balloon can be inflated with water, saline, or water-soluble contrast. The duration the inflated balloon should be held in position is not well-defined. It can vary from 30 seconds to 2 minutes. If fluoroscopy is being used, the balloon can be held in place until effacement of the waist is seen. Once the balloon is deflated, it should be withdrawn and the stricture site examined for mucosal tearing, and any complication including persistent bleeding or perforation. Adequate mucosal tearing (**Fig. 1**) indicates disruption of the mucosal layer of the gut lining, but not beyond the submucosal layer. If there is inadequate mucosal tearing, further dilation with the next larger balloon diameter should be carried out. It is not recommended to dilate more than 3 to 4 mm beyond the initial diameter of the stricture, especially if there is active inflammation at the site, unless there has been prior dilation of the same site to a higher diameter and it has now repeatedly scarred down. Even so, great

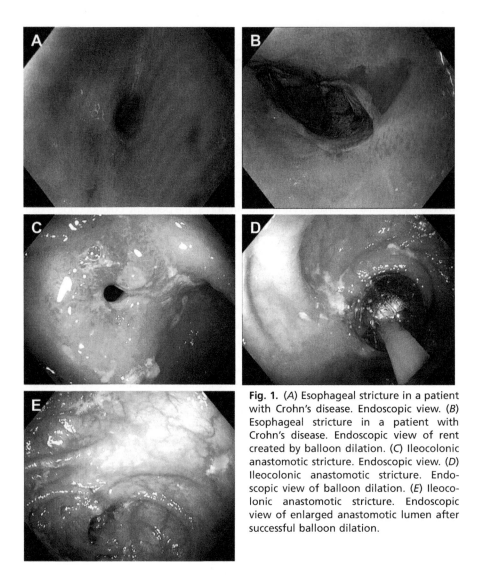

Fig. 1. (A) Esophageal stricture in a patient with Crohn's disease. Endoscopic view. (B) Esophageal stricture in a patient with Crohn's disease. Endoscopic view of rent created by balloon dilation. (C) Ileocolonic anastomotic stricture. Endoscopic view. (D) Ileocolonic anastomotic stricture. Endoscopic view of balloon dilation. (E) Ileocolonic anastomotic stricture. Endoscopic view of enlarged anastomotic lumen after successful balloon dilation.

caution should be used. Wire-guided hydrostatic dilation balloons (eg, CRE, Boston Scientific Corporation, Natick, MA) are also safer to use than non–wire-guided balloons, especially around angulated strictures, because they can guide the more distal tip of the balloon to remain within the bowel lumen and avoid perforation of the viscus wall beyond the stricture by the distal balloon tip. Another suggestion is to examine repeatedly the patient's abdomen to watch for distention, which may be a sign of a perforation. Maximal balloon diameter is usually 18 to 20 mm, although balloons as large as 25 mm have been described in studies. These larger diameter balloons have been associated with a definite higher risk of perforation without any evidence to suggest increased efficacy. Hence, we do not recommend dilating strictures to more than 18 to 20 mm.

Sixteen percent of patients undergoing ileal pouch–anal anastomoses develop stricturing at the pouch–anal site.[9] These strictures can be digitally dilated if they are soft and pliable. However, once they become more fibrotic, they can be dilated during endoscopy using either a graduated balloon as described above or Hegar's dilators, up to 18 mm in size.

Success of Endoscopic Balloon Dilation

Multiple studies over the years have documented the efficacy and safety of endoscopic balloon dilation in Crohn's disease strictures. One of the largest of these was published by Gustavsson and colleagues[10] in 2012. They reported the outcomes in 178 patients who underwent a total of 776 dilations. A stricture was defined as inability to pass the endoscope, and 81% of these patients were reported symptomatic. Eighty percent of the strictures were anastomotic (77% at an ileocolonic anastomosis). The maximal balloon dilation was 18 to 20 mm in the majority, but in 31% patients, a 25-mm balloon was used. Technical success was seen in 89%, with a complication rate of 5.3% (perforation was commonest). Of note, a significantly higher rate of complications (9.3%) was seen with use of the 25-mm balloon compared with 3.5% with balloons under 20 mm. Median follow-up time for a subset of 125 patients was 12 years. No further intervention or one additional dilation was needed in 80%, 57%, and 52% at 1, 3, and 5 years after the first dilation. Surgery-free survival did not differ between anastomotic versus de novo strictures.

The second largest study was published by Van Assche and colleagues[11] in 2010 where they reported the long-term efficacy of dilations in 138 patients followed for a median of 5.8 years; clinical results were robust and outweighed the risks of complications. Anastomotic strictures made up 84% of the cohort and ileal location was seen in 85%. All strictures were reported to be less than 5 cm in length, and a standard 16- to 18-mm balloon was used in all cases. The starting diameter of the strictures in the study was not described. This is a unique technique because usually we recommend starting dilation with a balloon that is slightly larger than the approximate stricture diameter, rather than using a standard diameter balloon for all strictures regardless of baseline lumen diameter. Immediate success rate of the dilation defined as ability to pass the colonoscope through the stricture was very high at 97.1%. No further dilation was needed in 54.3% of patients and 76.1% had no need for surgery after the first dilation. The complication rate was 5.1%, with 6 out of the 12 complications being perforation. It can be hypothesized that this complication rate could have been decreased if the starting balloon diameter was chosen based on the stricture diameter, rather than using a standard 18-mm balloon for all cases. Nevertheless, the success rate and surgery-free survival is impressive, and the authors also found that neither active disease nor medical therapy could predict the need for recurrent stricture dilation.

Atreja and colleagues[12] in 2014 reported outcomes in 128 patients with 169 Crohn's related strictures with a median follow-up of only 1.8 years. This cohort was unique because 52.1% of the strictures were de novo and only 47.9% were anastomotic. The median stricture length was 2 cm, and mean balloon size used was 16.6 mm. Active inflammation was seen in 60.1% of the strictures. Also unique was that 54.4% of these strictures could be traversed by the endoscope even before dilation. Redilation was performed in 58.6% patients, but the median number of redilations was only one. However, because the median follow-up was only 1.8 years, this study does not document long-term results. Complication rate was low at 3.1% per patient and only 0.93% per procedure, and 3 out of the 4 complications seen were perforations requiring surgical resection.

There have been 2 systematic reviews with metaanalyses published within the last year describing the efficacy of endoscopic balloon dilation for Crohn's disease strictures.[13,14] Morar and colleagues[13] included 25 studies with 1089 patients and 2664 dilations. Mean age at first dilation was 41 years. The follow-up times varied from a median minimum of 4 months to a median maximum of 83.5 months. Across 13 studies, 79.1% were anastomotic strictures and only 3.8% were upper GI strictures (but this was estimation because of missing data in 9 studies). A symptomatic response rate of 70.2% was shown but technical response was reported in 92.6% patients. No difference was seen on subgroup analyses between anastomotic versus de novo strictures or active versus quiescent inflammation at the stricture site, but there was heterogeneity in the reported data. The pooled complication rate was calculated at 6.4%, but perforation rate was 3%.

Navaneethan and colleagues[14] reported on 24 studies including 1163 patients with 1571 strictures. Mean age of the patients was similar; mean stricture length was 1 to 4 cm, and median follow-up time was 15 to 70 months. Ileocolonic anastomotic strictures were the majority (69%), and 31% were de novo strictures. Overall technical success was 89%. A single dilation was effective in 44% patients, and in 27%, surgical intervention was required either for failure of dilation or complication. Complication rate was found to be 4%, with perforation in 3%. Subanalyses showed that though success of endoscopic balloon dilation seems to be higher in anastomotic strictures compared with de novo strictures, this was not statistically significant. And, although only 5 studies had comparative data, they found a stricture length less than 4 cm had a significantly decreased risk of surgical intervention when compared with greater than 4 cm.

Krauss and colleagues[15] published an interesting and unique report in 2014 where they included 88 Crohn's disease patients with strictures and compared those with only endoscopic therapy, only surgical therapy, endoscopy followed by surgery and surgery followed by endoscopy. They found that endoscopic therapy was applied in 20 patients, of whom 9 required only a single dilation but the rest required up to 5 dilations. Stenoses in the surgical group had an average length of 6.5 cm compared with the endoscopic group which was 3.0 cm. Endoscopic balloon dilation also worked more effectively in fibrotic strictures, which were shorter (mean, 4.0 cm) than inflammatory strictures (mean length, 7.5 cm). In the surgical group, 35% developed new stenoses, of which 75% were treated with endoscopic balloon dilation. Also, smoking was found to be a risk factor for recurrent stenosis.

A recent study by Sunada and colleagues[16] reports on the long-term outcomes of 321 double balloon enteroscopy-assisted dilations of Crohn's strictures in 85 patients. Seventy-one percent were antegrade enteroscopies, the mean balloon diameter at first dilation was 12.4 mm, mean follow-up period was 41.9 months, and surgery-free rate after the initial double balloon enteroscopy-assisted endoscopic balloon dilation was 87.3% at 1 year, 78.1% at 3 years, and 74.2% at 5 years. Complication rate was 1% overall and perforation rate was 0.8% per procedure and 4.7% per patient.

The success of endoscopic dilation of ileal pouch–anal anastomosis strictures was published in a report by Shen and colleagues[17] where 646 strictures in 150 patients were dilated during 406 pouchoscopies. Median stricture length was 1 cm and median balloon size was 20 mm. Two perforations occurred. In a median follow-up period of 9.6 years, 87.3% patients were able to retain their pouches.

Other Adjunctive Techniques

Intralesional injection of a long-acting corticosteroid has been used as an adjunct to endoscopic balloon dilation to help maintain the efficacy of the dilation owing to a proposed local antiinflammatory effect. The most commonly used agent is triamcinolone, which is injected in a dose from 40 to 100 mg usually in 4 to 5 aliquots at different sites within the stricture. This injection is performed after maximal dilation. The data regarding the efficacy of intralesional steroid injection is conflicting. Some studies[12,18] did not find any beneficial effects but other small studies[19–22] suggested a favorable effect of prolonging the need for further dilation or surgery. Similarly, 2 small case series have described the use of intralesional infliximab to treat strictures, but these data are not robust enough to support widespread use of the agent in this application.[23,24]

Another adjunctive treatment modality for strictures is needle-knife strictureplasty, wherein a needle-knife from the pancreaticobiliary endoscopy armamentarium is used as an adjunctive technique to perform multisite monopolar electroincision of refractory fibrotic strictures. However, this technique has only been described in a few case reports and should not be performed routinely owing to high risk of perforation[25,26] Self-expanding stents have been reported in a few recent studies as an alternative to repeated Endoscopic balloon dilation of strictures in Crohn's disease. These have included both fully covered metallic stents[27–29] and biodegradable stents.[30] They have had reasonable success rates in delaying the need for surgery, but have high migration rates. Hence, these are not yet recommended for routine use.

In conclusion, endoscopic balloon dilation is a safe and efficacious therapy for luminal strictures in inflammatory bowel disease and should be used to treat symptoms and prevent future morbidity.

BILIARY STRICTURE MANAGEMENT IN PRIMARY SCLEROSING CHOLANGITIS

PSC is an idiopathic, chronic inflammatory disorder that leads to fibrosis and multifocal structuring of the bile ducts. Chronic obstruction of the bile ducts ensues, leading to complications including recurrent episodes of bacterial cholangitis, and to biliary cirrhosis with its associated portal hypertensive stigmata and hepatic synthetic dysfunction. PSC also confers an increased risk of cholangiocarcinoma (CCA); approximately 5% of patients with PSC-IBD will develop CCA compared with less than 0.1% of IBD patients without PSC resulting in a 55-fold greater risk of this otherwise uncommon malignancy.[31] Liver transplantation is the only curative treatment, but PSC can recur after transplantation in 10% of patients.[32,33]

PSC is strongly associated with inflammatory bowel disease (IBD). The vast majority—67% to 73%—of patients with PSC have IBD.[34,35] The stronger association is with ulcerative colitis as opposed to Crohn's disease. Conversely, PSC itself is an uncommon disorder, even in the presence of IBD: only 3% of patients with IBD develop PSC.[36]

Endoscopy, in the form of ERCP, plays a central role in the diagnosis and management of PSC.[37] Liver biopsy has limited sensitivity in the diagnosis of PSC, because many of the histologic features seen in this disorder are nonspecific, and the hallmark finding of periductal lamellar fibrosis is infrequently detected. Thus, before the advent of MR cholangiopancreatography (MRCP), ERCP was the diagnostic study of first choice when an individual presenting with cholestatic symptoms or liver enzyme elevations—particularly a patient with IBD—required bile duct imaging to determine if the patient had developed PSC. The introduction of MRCP was revolutionary in the diagnostic workup of PSC, permitting cholangiographic imaging without the risks inherent to ERCP but with comparable sensitivity and specificity. This has led to MRCP having largely supplanted ERCP as the initial imaging study in the primary diagnosis of PSC, reserving ERCP for use as a confirmatory study.[38–40]

Obtaining a good cholangiogram when ERCP is performed in a patient with PSC requires extra care and effort on the part of the endoscopist. Biliary strictures resulting from PSC contribute to compromised drainage of contrast injected during ERCP. Thus, preprocedure and postprocedure antibiotics are recommended by many experts and guidelines to reduce the risk of procedure-induced cholangitis.[41] Strictures upstream from the cystic duct insertion are common, and the gradient to contrast flow antegrade across the stricture is often higher than the flow gradient through the cystic duct into the gallbladder, leading to undesirable excessive contrast filling of the gallbladder, leading to gallbladder distention and associated patient discomfort, as well as poor or incomplete opacification of the biliary tree upstream from the cystic duct insertion. To prevent such unwanted contrast diversion away from the more proximal biliary tree, a stone extraction balloon catheter is often used to undertake the contrast cholangiogram in the setting of PSC. By inflating the balloon proximal to the cystic duct insertion, then injection contrast slowly against the balloon, contrast is forced upstream, across the higher flow gradients posed by the strictures upstream. This leads to fuller opacification of the biliary tree to the periphery of the ducts, and also reduces retrograde escape of contrast into the cystic duct and gallbladder (**Fig. 2**). Some strictures may be so tight that even balloon occlusion cholangiography does not net opacification of the entire biliary tree. Comparison with MRCP images will demonstrate which ducts have not been opacified successfully at ERCP, because such duct systems frequently involve prestenotic dilatation of ducts upstream from the tight stricture. Such dilatation typically appears prominently on MRCP, because imaging in MRI depends on the bile naturally occupying the duct lumen, as opposed to ERCP, which depends on the retrograde flow of contrast across the stricture into the duct lumen upstream from the stricture.[42]

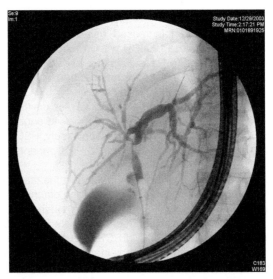

Fig. 2. Balloon occlusion cholangiogram of patient with primary sclerosing cholangitis of the intrahepatic ducts with hilar dominant stricture and prestenotic dilatation of left intrahepatic ducts; fluoroscopic view.

Today, the main roles of ERCP in PSC consist of tissue acquisition and therapeutic intervention. Given the increased risk of CCA in PSC, the identification on MRCP of a dominant stricture or other duct stigmata suspicious for the development of CCA will trigger a request for intraductal brushings or biopsies to obtain tissue specimens for cytologic or histologic examination. In the patient with PSC who develops symptomatic biliary obstruction with jaundice, pruritus, or ascending cholangitis, ERCP can offer robust therapeutic interventions to overcome duct obstruction and its various complications.

DIAGNOSTIC TISSUE ACQUISITION IN PRIMARY SCLEROSING CHOLANGITIS

Tissue acquisition at ERCP to exclude CCA in PSC is undertaken using 3 major techniques: brush cytology, transpapillary intraductal forceps biopsy, and choledochoscopically guided (cholangioscopically guided) miniature forceps biopsy. The most often relied upon, and best-studied, method is that of intraductal brush cytology. After a guidewire has been positioned across the segment of duct to be sampled, a Papanicolaou-type cytology brush is advanced through the duodenoscope over the guidewire. The brush is then advanced and withdrawn, back and forth multiple times, across the targeted stricture in the duct in a reciprocating fashion, then retracted back into its catheter before being removed from the scope (**Fig. 3**). It is then placed in a preservative solution to be delivered to the cytology laboratory for processing. The technique of brush cytology applied to bile duct strictures is encumbered by notoriously low sensitivity, with most studies demonstrating values of 50% to 60%.[43–45] As a result, additional effort is often invested to improve diagnostic yield. Some studies demonstrate that dilation of the stricture before brushing improves cytologic and diagnostic yield, but others do not.[46–48] Augmenting brush cytology with at least 1 additional method of tissue acquisition has also been demonstrated to improve

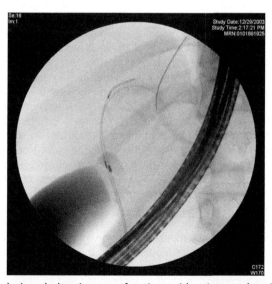

Fig. 3. Balloon occlusion cholangiogram of patient with primary sclerosing cholangitis of the intrahepatic ducts with hilar dominant stricture and prestenotic dilatation of left intrahepatic ducts; fluoroscopic view of wire-guided brush cytology of dominant hilar biliary stricture.

sensitivity.[49] The most common adjunctive modality is transpapillary intraductal forceps biopsy, typically performed with a regular biopsy forceps, or a smaller variety such as a pediatric or dedicated intraductal forceps, available in various proprietary iterations. After cholangiography and dilation with brush cytology, the forceps is introduced carefully up the bile duct under fluoroscopic guidance to the stricture where biopsies are obtained. Some studies suggest adding intraductal forceps biopsy improves sensitivity by 10% to 20% over brushing alone, but others demonstrate more modest gains.[50] Although, historically, fine needle aspiration has been another available adjunctive intraductal tissue-acquisitive modality, it has been largely abandoned over the past decade or more as intraductal forceps, which generally provide a larger specimen, have become increasingly popular and the technique widely practiced.[51,52] Intraductal forceps biopsy can also be performed via a transcholedochoscopic approach. In this method, a miniature choledochoscope is advanced through the accessory channel of the duodenoscope, typically over a guidewire that has already been positioned in the bile duct. The choledochoscope is then advanced up the bile duct under direct choledochoscopic view and simultaneous fluoroscopic guidance, and the area of the stricture directly visualized by the choledochoscope. A dedicated miniature forceps is then advanced through the accessory channel of the choledochoscope to biopsy the desired area of the duct directly.[53] Some studies demonstrate that this technique can increase sensitivity by 10% to 20% above brushing alone, although others suggest a more modest additional diagnostic impact.[54] It is not completely clear whether choledochoscopically guided intraductal biopsy consistently delivers higher incremental diagnostic yield than direct intraductal forceps biopsy; some studies have suggested this but others have not.[55–57] The only choledochoscope presently available commercially is a one-time use device that accepts only a proprietary miniature forceps, which is also a 1-time use device. Thus, the use of this particular method can add substantially to procedure cost, and, thus, is often reserved for use when other methods have failed to establish a diagnosis or when direct choledochoscopic visualization might provide diagnostic benefit beyond simply providing a conduit for intraductal biopsy forceps. Non–fiber-optic, video cholangioscopes in reusable, multiuse platforms have been developed but are presently available only for investigational use.[58,59] These devices are being developed in both transduodenoscopic and direct per-oral cholangioscope platforms. Many groups have described the use of small-caliber endoscopes as direct per-oral cholangioscopes in patients whose duodenal anatomy and bile duct diameter will accommodate this caliber of direct access bile duct endoscopy, including use of an adjunctive intraductal balloon catheter and overtube to improve duct access and scope stability.[60–64] Other intraductal imaging modalities and advanced imaging technologies, such as intraductal probe ultrasound, probe-based confocal endomicroscopy, and optical coherence tomography have demonstrated the ability to provide enhanced imaging data in the evaluation of biliary strictures, but their roles remain largely investigational, and their application in standard clinical practice is, as yet, incompletely defined. These imaging technologies exist as a probe-based platform. As such, because the imaging probe itself is advanced into the bile duct through the accessory channel of the duodenoscope, none of these modalities is able to provide for real-time visual guidance of biopsies using the image delivered by the probe-based instrument itself.[65–68]

ERCP fine-needle aspiration is another technique used to obtain cytologic specimens at ERCP. A dedicated needle catheter is advanced through the duodenoscope into the bile duct under fluoroscopic guidance, and then negative pressure is applied while the needle is targeted into the stricture or lesion of interest to obtain a cytologic or tissue specimen.[52] This technique was largely supplanted by transpapillary intraductal forceps biopsy and, in some instances of distal common bile duct strictures, by endoscopic ultrasound-guided fine-needle aspiration.[69]

Because even the addition of a second tissue acquisitive modality leaves sensitivity substantially below 90%, advanced cytologic methods are sometimes used to increase diagnostic sensitivity beyond that of cytology and histology alone. Fluorescence in situ hybridization is the most prevalent such technique to detect aneuploidy, a characteristic of malignancy, in biliary cytology specimens. In this method, cells obtained for cytology are analyzed for chromosomal abnormalities in their DNA (**Fig. 4**). The assay detects various aneuploidies and polysomies; polysomy seems to be the most sensitive and specific for CCA, particularly if multifocal. Overall, fluorescence in situ hybridization added to optical cytology increases sensitivity and overall diagnostic yield while minimally impacting specificity, which is amply high even with cytology alone.[70–72] Another postprocessing method is digital image analysis, in which aneuploidy is inferred through quantitation of DNA via microscopic visualization of dye-stained nuclei.[42,73] Various biomarkers are under active investigation to enhance the diagnostic capabilities of endoscopy in the detection of CCA in the setting of PSC.[74,75]

THERAPEUTIC ROLE IN PRIMARY SCLEROSING CHOLANGITIS

The role of ERCP in therapeutic intervention for PSC is focused on relief of biliary obstructive symptoms, such as jaundice and pruritus, and upon treatment of bacterial cholangitis attributable to biliary obstruction. In PSC, such obstruction results primarily from benign, fibroinflammatory stricture formation in the bile duct, but may also involve bile duct stones and sludge, as well as other biliary debris. ERCP can relieve

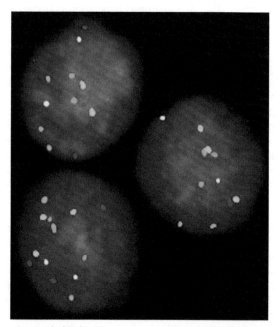

Fig. 4. Fluorescence in situ hybridization assay consistent with malignancy. (*Courtesy of* Dr. Michael J. Levy, Mayo Clinic Foundation, Rochester, MN; with permission.)

such obstruction through stricture dilation, and, in selected cases, through temporary stent placement. In cases where CCA or hepatocellular carcinoma develop, malignant strictures may obstruct the bile duct, resulting not only in cholestatic symptoms, but also potentially limiting the administration of chemotherapeutic agents that cannot be administered when cholestasis limits the biliary excretion of their toxic metabolic products. In these patients, ERCP may relieve biliary obstruction through stricture dilation, placement of temporary or permanent stents, or ablative therapies such as photodynamic therapy or radiofrequency ablation.[76] ERCP can also provide a conduit for the placement of radioactive seeds by inserting nasobiliary drains, which facilitate brachytherapy administration.[77]

Stricture Dilation

Stricture dilation in PSC is undertaken for 2 reasons: to relieve symptoms associated with bile duct obstructions, such as jaundice, ascending cholangitis, and pruritus, and to facilitate brush cytology, intraductal biopsy, and clearance of stones and other debris, and its effectiveness demonstrated in multiple series spanning over 2 decades.[78,79] Stricture dilation is generally technically easier in the extrahepatic, compared with the intrahepatic, bile ducts. At and above the hilum, stricture dilation can be a considerably more complex undertaking, because obtaining guidewire access to a particular branch bile duct, or biliary radicle, requires additional skill, effort, and time, and also because the decision to place a stent postdilation often obligates the endoscopist to consider whether placement of a solid-walled endoprosthesis might impede, or even obstruct, the flow of an adjacent, confluent, or contralateral duct (so-called jailing of a duct or radicle), leading to reduced sectoral bile flow, localized cholangitis, or liver abscess.

There are several types of dilators available for use in the bile duct. The most commonly used is the hydrostatic dilation balloon, which, in the bile duct, is always of the wire-guided variety (**Fig. 5**). Controlled expansion is undertaken under fluoroscopic guidance using a manometric inflation device filled with water-soluble radiologic contrast identical to that used for the ERCP cholangiogram. Balloon diameter is chosen based on the native diameter of the duct, typically selecting a diameter incrementally larger than native duct diameter. The balloon is inflated under fluoroscopic guidance until the waist created where the stricture impacts the balloon is obliterated or until the balloon reaches its specified burst pressure, whichever is attained first. Longer strictures can be dilated with multiple inflations of the balloon applied sequentially along the axis of the stricture. The advantages of a balloon dilator over a passage, or tapered-catheter dilatator, include larger available diameters, multiple diameters in 1 balloon based on inflation pressure, full dilation force conferred radially, ability to visualize fluoroscopically a waist at the stricture site, and capability to view and confirm waist obliteration fluoroscopically, in real time, as a surrogate marker for dilation effectiveness.

A passage, or coaxial, dilator may also be used, usually for smaller ducts, or when a stricture is too tight to allow initial traversal with a dilation balloon. This type of dilator is a plastic catheter that has a gentle taper to it, beginning with a tip that is typically as narrow as the guidewire used with it permits. The point at which the taper ends, and full catheter diameter is attained, is often demarcated with a radiopaque marker such as a metal ring (**Fig. 6**). These come in various sizes, with the smallest tapered end measuring 3 Fr, and the largest diameter at the top end of the taper measuring 11.5 Fr, which corresponds with the largest diameter instrument that can traverse the accessory channel of a therapeutic duodenoscope. The advantages of a passage dilator include a narrower minimal diameter of the smallest dilation catheter available as compared with the smallest obtainable low-profile dilation balloon, the possibility that the shear component of the force applied to the dilator may lead to increased slough of cells and tissue at the site of a stricture and increase cytologic yield of subsequent brushing or biopsy, and lower per-unit cost.

If a stricture is too tight to allow guidewire access across it, endoscopic dilation cannot be performed. In this situation, when clinically required—usually for drainage rather than tissue acquisition alone—percutaneous access in interventional radiology, or EUS-assisted approaches, can provide rendezvous access. In this technique, needle puncture of the duct upstream from the stricture is undertaken via percutaneous transhepatic cholangiography or EUS, and a guidewire inserted antegrade across the stricture. In the percutaneous method, a temporary catheter (external drain) may be inserted over the guidewire. The duodenoscope is then positioned in the duodenal sweep, and the guidewire placed in interventional radiology (IR) or at EUS is then grasped with a snare, brought retrograde through the accessory channel of the duodenoscope, and used as the access wire for subsequent ERCP maneuvers including any additional stricture dilation needed, tissue acquisition, and stent insertion.[80–82]

Stenting

Traditional biliary stents are tubular plastic devices that are typically 7 to 11.5 Fr in diameter, 3 to 18 cm in length, and come in a number of different configurations including shapes, profiles, and presence or absence of sidewall fenestrations. Most are made of polyethylene, but some silicone-elastic and polytetrafluoroethylene (Teflon) iterations are also available. The maximal diameter of a single plastic stent is limited by the luminal diameter of the accessory channel of the duodenoscope through which it is deployed. However, larger diameter stenting can be accomplished by inserting 2 or more plastic stents in a parallel fashion using the concept of aggregate stenting, to yield an aggregate stent diameter. Individual stents with a diameter greater than that of the lumen of the duodenoscope accessory channel are available in the form of a self-expanding metallic biliary stents, and these are described in greater detail below. The vast majority of stents used to treat PSC are of the plastic variety—temporary and fully removable.

Stent placement in the setting of PSC has long been an area of controversy and empiric approach.[83] Strong, definitive, high-quality data on this topic has been difficult to generate for a number of reasons, including not only the relative rarity of the disorder, but also both the heterogeneity of disease presentation in PSC and the variation in foci of stricture involvement superimposed on highly variable duct anatomy. Strictures requiring dilation and stenting also are generally not accompanied by normal ducts upstream; more proximally located ducts are also involved with strictures and irregularities. Such upstream ducts also sometimes contain stasis stones, sludge, or both, which can contribute to flow obstruction as well as serve as a nidus for bacterial colonization and infection. In such a setting, a stent placed across the dominant stricture downstream may serve as a conduit to convey retrograde flow of duodenal contents, including food debris and enteric bacteria, up into these more proximal ducts, where outflow of such refluxed material is compromised, by definition, by the strictures and irregularities present in these diseased peripheral bile ducts.

No randomized controlled trials assessing the effect of postdilation stenting of biliary strictures in PSC are available to guide decision making in this realm. Most data on this topic come from retrospective reviews and observational studies of small groups of patients. Strictures in the setting of PSC differ from other benign biliary strictures, such as those resulting from anastomotic fibrosis or chronic pancreatitis, because, in the vast majority of such studies in non-PSC patients, the ducts upstream

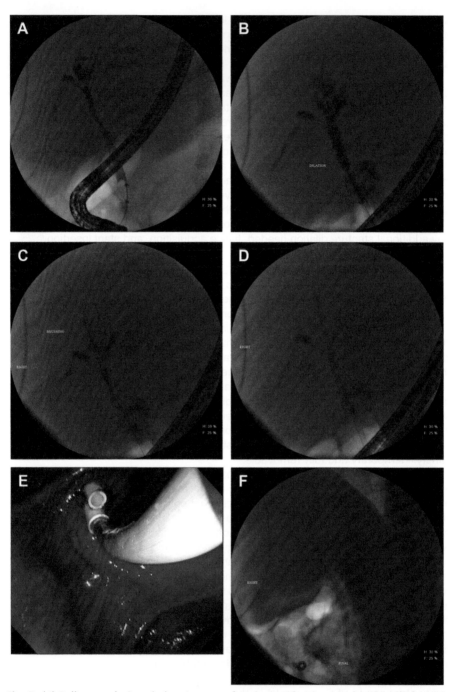

Fig. 5. (*A*) Balloon occlusion cholangiogram of patient with primary sclerosing cholangitis of the intrahepatic ducts with hilar dominant stricture and upstream prestenotic ductal dilatation of intrahepatic ducts; fluoroscopic view of guidewire looping at tight stricture. (*B*) Balloon occlusion cholangiogram of patient with primary sclerosing cholangitis of the intrahepatic ducts with hilar-dominant stricture and upstream prestenotic ductal dilatation of

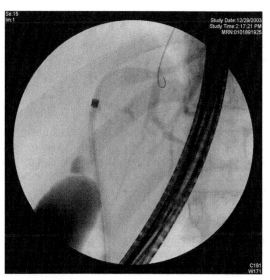

Fig. 6. Passage (coaxial) dilation of dominant hilar biliary stricture in patient with primary sclerosing cholangitis; fluoroscopic view.

from the stricture are normal. In contradistinction, the risk-to-benefit proposal in stenting differs in PSC, where the stricture to be addressed is typically not the only duct abnormality or requiring consideration. A number of studies have suggested benefit of stent placement after dilation of dominant strictures in PSC (see **Fig. 5**). However, others have demonstrated the added risks incurred in placing stents as compared with dilation alone. Studies taking into account the impact of duration of stent therapy tend to suggest that, if stenting is undertaken after dilation in PSC, that the stent should remain in situ for only a short duration in most circumstances. Many experts first try dilation alone, and only if the desired results—such as resolution of jaundice, mitigation of recurrent episodes of bacterial cholangitis, or improvement of pruritus—are not achieved, then pursue short-term postdilation stenting, typically for 1 to 3 weeks.[79,84–87]

Biliary self-expanding metallic stents (SEMS) come in 3 varieties: bare metal, or uncovered (U-SEMS), partially covered (PC-SEMS), and fully covered (FC-SEMS). Both U-SEMS and PC-SEMS become permanently embedded in biliary tissue and are not

---

intrahepatic ducts; fluoroscopic view of balloon dilation of hilar dominant stricture. (*C*) Balloon occlusion cholangiogram of patient with primary sclerosing cholangitis of the intrahepatic ducts with hilar dominant stricture and upstream prestenotic ductal dilatation of intrahepatic ducts; fluoroscopic view of balloon dilation of hilar dominant stricture. (*D*) Balloon occlusion cholangiogram of patient with primary sclerosing cholangitis of the intrahepatic ducts with hilar dominant stricture and upstream prestenotic ductal dilatation of intrahepatic ducts. Fluoroscopic view of stent placement after balloon dilation of hilar dominant stricture. (*E*) Insertion of second biliary stent parallel to initially inserted stent. Endoscopic view. (*F*) Balloon occlusion cholangiogram of patient with primary sclerosing cholangitis of the intrahepatic ducts with hilar dominant stricture and upstream prestenotic ductal dilatation of intrahepatic ducts. Fluoroscopic view of second stent placed parallel to initial stent across hilar dominant stricture.

considered to be removable after implantation. As a result, they are reserved for malignant biliary obstruction without expectation of removability, and generally not appropriate for deployment in patients with benign conditions such as PSC. FC-SEMS stents have a closed wall design, where the entire metal mesh stent is covered in a silicone or polytetrafluoroethylene membrane including the interstices between the wires, thus preventing them from embedding themselves in the wall of the bile duct. Although they are approved by the US Food ad Drug Administration for use in malignant biliary strictures, they are widely used off-label for the treatment of various benign strictures. Given their combined characteristics of being both expansile and solid-walled, however, FC-SEMS are generally considered not to be indicated for use at or above the hilum. Although FC-SEMS use in PSC has been described, no data beyond case reports and small series is available, and the role of these devices in PSC remains largely undetermined.[88–91]

SUMMARY

General gastroenterologists, IBD specialists and advanced endoscopists all play a role in treating patients with IBD. For patients with Crohn's disease-related strictures at either native intestine or an anastomosis, dilation with balloons can be safely accomplished. Repeat dilation may be required but the risk of perforation is acceptably low if patients are optimally medically managed to reduce the inflammation at the site. Biliary strictures in PSC are more complex requiring advanced endoscopy techniques to be certain that malignancy is not present and to treat the stricture endoscopically.

REFERENCES

1. Cosnes J, Cattan S, Blain A, et al. Long-term evolution of disease behavior of Crohn's disease. Inflamm Bowel Dis 2002;8(4):244–50.
2. Rieder F, Zimmermann EM, Remzi FH, et al. Crohn's disease complicated by strictures: a systematic review. Gut 2013;62(7):1072–84.
3. Peyrin-Biroulet L, Loftus EV Jr, Colombel JF, et al. The natural history of adult Crohn's disease in population-based cohorts. Am J Gastroenterol 2010;105(2): 289–97.
4. Bernstein CN, Ng SC, Lakatos PL, et al. A review of mortality and surgery in ulcerative colitis: milestones of the seriousness of the disease. Inflamm Bowel Dis 2013;19(9):2001–10.
5. Longobardi T, Bernstein CN. Health care resource utilization in inflammatory bowel disease. Clin Gastroenterol Hepatol 2006;4(6):731–43.
6. Samuel S, Ingle SB, Dhillon S, et al. Cumulative incidence and risk factors for hospitalization and surgery in a population-based cohort of ulcerative colitis. Inflamm Bowel Dis 2013;19(9):1858–66.
7. Solberg IC, Lygren I, Jahnsen J, et al. Clinical course during the first 10 years of ulcerative colitis: results from a population-based inception cohort (IBSEN Study). Scand J Gastroenterol 2009;44(4):431–40.
8. Bruining DH, Bhatnagar G, Rimola J, et al. CT and MR enterography in Crohn's disease: current and future applications. Abdom Imaging 2015;40(5):965–74.
9. Lewis WG, Kuzu A, Sagar PM, et al. Stricture at the pouch-anal anastomosis after restorative proctocolectomy. Dis Colon Rectum 1994;37(2):120–5.
10. Gustavsson A, Magnuson A, Blomberg B, et al. Endoscopic dilation is an efficacious and safe treatment of intestinal strictures in Crohn's disease. Aliment Pharmacol Ther 2012;36(2):151–8.

11. Thienpont C, D'Hoore A, Vermeire S, et al. Long-term outcome of endoscopic dilatation in patients with Crohn's disease is not affected by disease activity or medical therapy. Gut 2010;59(3):320–4.

12. Atreja A, Aggarwal A, Dwivedi S, et al. Safety and efficacy of endoscopic dilation for primary and anastomotic Crohn's disease strictures. J Crohns Colitis 2014; 8(5):392–400.

13. Morar PS, Faiz O, Warusavitarne J, et al. Systematic review with meta-analysis: endoscopic balloon dilatation for Crohn's disease strictures. Aliment Pharmacol Ther 2015;42(10):1137–48.

14. Navaneethan U, Lourdusamy V, Njei B, et al. Endoscopic balloon dilation in the management of strictures in Crohn's disease: a systematic review and meta-analysis of non-randomized trials. Surg Endosc 2016. [Epub ahead of print].

15. Krauss E, Agaimy A, Gottfried A, et al. Long term follow up of through-the-scope balloon dilation as compared to strictureplasty and bowel resection of intestinal strictures in Crohn's disease. Int J Clin Exp Pathol 2014;7(11):7419–31.

16. Sunada K, Shinozaki S, Nagayama M, et al. Long-term outcomes in patients with small intestinal strictures secondary to Crohn's disease after double-balloon endoscopy-assisted balloon dilation. Inflamm Bowel Dis 2016;22(2):380–6.

17. Shen B, Lian L, Kiran RP, et al. Efficacy and safety of endoscopic treatment of ileal pouch strictures. Inflamm Bowel Dis 2011;17(12):2527–35.

18. East JE, Brooker JC, Rutter MD, et al. A pilot study of intrastricture steroid versus placebo injection after balloon dilatation of Crohn's strictures. Clin Gastroenterol Hepatol 2007;5(9):1065–9.

19. Brooker JC, Beckett CG, Saunders BP, et al. Long-acting steroid injection after endoscopic dilation of anastomotic Crohn's strictures may improve the outcome: a retrospective case series. Endoscopy 2003;35(4):333–7.

20. Di Nardo G, Oliva S, Passariello M, et al. Intralesional steroid injection after endoscopic balloon dilation in pediatric Crohn's disease with stricture: a prospective, randomized, double-blind, controlled trial. Gastrointest Endosc 2010;72(6): 1201–8.

21. Ramboer C, Verhamme M, Dhondt E, et al. Endoscopic treatment of stenosis in recurrent Crohn's disease with balloon dilation combined with local corticosteroid injection. Gastrointest Endosc 1995;42(3):252–5.

22. Singh VV, Draganov P, Valentine J. Efficacy and safety of endoscopic balloon dilation of symptomatic upper and lower gastrointestinal Crohn's disease strictures. J Clin Gastroenterol 2005;39(4):284–90.

23. Hendel J, Karstensen JG, Vilmann P. Serial intralesional injections of infliximab in small bowel Crohn's strictures are feasible and might lower inflammation. United European Gastroenterol J 2014;2(5):406–12.

24. Swaminath A, Lichtiger S. Dilation of colonic strictures by intralesional injection of infliximab in patients with Crohn's colitis. Inflamm Bowel Dis 2008;14(2):213–6.

25. Chen M, Shen B. Endoscopic needle-knife stricturotomy for nipple valve stricture of continent ileostomy (with video). Gastrointest Endosc 2015;81(5):1287–8 [discussion: 1288–9].

26. Kerkhof M, Dewint P, Koch AD, et al. Endoscopic needle-knife treatment of refractory ileo-ascending anastomotic stricture. Endoscopy 2013;45(Suppl 2 UCTN): E57–8.

27. Attar A, Maunoury V, Vahedi K, et al. Safety and efficacy of extractible self-expandable metal stents in the treatment of Crohn's disease intestinal strictures: a prospective pilot study. Inflamm Bowel Dis 2012;18(10):1849–54.

28. Branche J, Attar A, Vernier-Massouille G, et al. Extractible self-expandable metal stent in the treatment of Crohn's disease anastomotic strictures. Endoscopy 2012; 44(Suppl 2 UCTN):E325–6.

29. Levine RA, Wasvary H, Kadro O. Endoprosthetic management of refractory ileocolonic anastomotic strictures after resection for Crohn's disease: report of nine-year follow-up and review of the literature. Inflamm Bowel Dis 2012;18(3):506–12.

30. Rejchrt S, Kopacova M, Brozik J, et al. Biodegradable stents for the treatment of benign stenoses of the small and large intestines. Endoscopy 2011;43(10): 911–7.

31. Ananthakrishnan AN, Cagan A, Gainer VS, et al. Mortality and extraintestinal cancers in patients with primary sclerosing cholangitis and inflammatory bowel disease. J Crohns Colitis 2014;8(9):956–63.

32. Graziadei IW, Wisner RH, Batts KP, et al. Recurrence of primary sclerosing cholangitis following liver transplantation. Hepatology 1999;29(4):1050–6.

33. Silveira MG, Lindor KD. Primary sclerosing cholangitis. Can J Gastroenterol 2008; 22(8):689–98.

34. Gulamhusein AF, Eaton JE, Tabibian JH, et al. Duration of inflammatory bowel disease is associated with increased risk of cholangiocarcinoma in patients with primary sclerosing cholangitis and IBD. Am J Gastroenterol 2016;111(5):705–11.

35. Boonstra K, van Erpecum KJ, van Nieuwkerk KM, et al. Primary sclerosing cholangitis is associated with a distinct phenotype of inflammatory bowel disease. Inflamm Bowel Dis 2012;18(12):2270–6.

36. Ponsioen CY. Diagnosis, differential diagnosis, and epidemiology of primary sclerosing cholangitis. Dig Dis 2015;33(Suppl 2):134–9.

37. Martin JA. Endoscopic management of primary sclerosing cholangitis: state of the art. Am J Gastroenterol 2007;102:S32–7.

38. Talwalkar JA, Angulo P, Johnson CD, et al. Cost-minimization analysis of MRC versus ERCP for the diagnosis of primary sclerosing cholangitis. Hepatology 2004;40(1):39–45.

39. Meagher S, Yusoff I, Kennedy W, et al. The roles of magnetic resonance and endoscopic retrograde cholangiopancreatography (MRCP and ERCP) in the diagnosis of patients with suspected sclerosing cholangitis: a cost-effectiveness analysis. Endoscopy 2007;39(3):222–8.

40. Weber C, Kuhlencordt R, Grotelueschen R, et al. Magnetic resonance cholangiopancreatography in the diagnosis of primary sclerosing cholangitis. Endoscopy 2008;40(9):739–45.

41. ASGE Standards of Practice Committee, Khashab MA, Chithadi KV, et al. Antibiotic prophylaxis for GI endoscopy. Gastrointest Endosc 2015;81(1):81–9.

42. Berstad AE, Aabakken L, Smith HJ, et al. Diagnostic accuracy of magnetic resonance and endoscopic retrograde cholangiography in primary sclerosing cholangitis. Clin Gastroenterol Hepatol 2006;4(4):514–20.

43. Trikudanathan G, Navaneethan U, Njei B, et al. Diagnostic yield of bile duct brushings for cholangiocarcinoma in primary sclerosing cholangitis: a systematic review and meta-analysis. Gastrointest Endosc 2014;79(5):783–9.

44. Baskin-Bey ES, Moreno Luna LE, Gores GJ. Diagnosis of cholangiocarcinoma in patients with PSC: a sight on cytology. J Hepatol 2006;45(4):476–9.

45. Boberg KM, Jebsen P, Clausen OP, et al. Diagnostic benefit of biliary brush cytology in cholangiocarcinoma in primary sclerosing cholangitis. J Hepatol 2006;45:568–74.

46. Fogel EL, Sherman S, Devereaux B, et al. Does stricture dilation add to the yield of brush cytology in the evaluation of malignant biliary obstruction? Am J Gastroenterol 2000;95:2477.

47. de Bellis M, Fogel EL, Sherman S, et al. Influence of stricture dilation and repeat brushing on the cancer detection rate of brush cytology in the evaluation of malignant biliary obstruction. Gastrointest Endosc 2003;58(2):176–82.

48. Ornellas LC, Santos Gda C, Nakao FS, et al. Comparison between endoscopic brush cytology performed before and after biliary stricture dilation for cancer detection. Arq Gastroenterol 2006;43(1):20–3.

49. Nanda A, Brown JM, Berger SH, et al. Triple modality testing by endoscopic retrograde cholangiopancreatography for the diagnosis of cholangiocarcinoma. Therap Adv Gastroenterol 2015;8(2):56–65.

50. Navaneethan U, Njei B, Lourdusamy V, et al. Comparative effectiveness of biliary brush cytology and intraductal biopsy for detection of malignant biliary strictures: a systematic review and meta-analysis. Gastrointest Endosc 2015;81(1):168–76.

51. Lee SJ, Lee YS, Lee MG, et al. Triple-tissue sampling during endoscopic retrograde cholangiopancreatography increases the overall diagnostic sensitivity for cholangiocarcinoma. Gut Liver 2014;8(6):669–73.

52. Farrell RJ, Jain AK, Brandwein SL, et al. The combination of stricture dilation, endoscopic needle aspiration, and biliary brushings significantly improves diagnostic yield from malignant bile duct strictures. Gastrointest Endosc 2001;54(5):587–94.

53. Kurihara T, Yasuda I, Isayama H, et al. Diagnostic and therapeutic single-operator cholangiopancreatoscopy in biliopancreatic diseases: prospective multicenter study in Japan. World J Gastroenterol 2016;22(5):1891–901.

54. Navaneethan U, Hasan MK, Lourdusamy V, et al. Single-operator cholangioscopy and targeted biopsies in the diagnosis of indeterminate biliary strictures: a systematic review. Gastrointest Endosc 2015;82(4):608–14.

55. Walter D, Peveling-Oberhag J, Schulze F, et al. Intraductal biopsies in indeterminate biliary stricture: Evaluation of histopathological criteria in fluoroscopy- vs. cholangioscopy guided technique. Dig Liver Dis 2016;48(7):765–70.

56. Draganov PV, Chauhan S, Wagh MS, et al. Diagnostic accuracy of conventional and cholangioscopy-guided sampling of indeterminate biliary lesions at the time of ERCP: a prospective, long-term follow-up study. Gastrointest Endosc 2012;75(2):347–53.

57. Hartman DJ, Slivka A, Giusto DA, et al. Tissue yield and diagnostic efficacy of fluoroscopic and cholangioscopic techniques to assess indeterminate biliary strictures. Clin Gastroenterol Hepatol 2012;10(9):1042–6.

58. Shah RJ. Innovations in intraductal endoscopy: cholangioscopy and pancreatoscopy. Gastrointest Endosc Clin N Am 2015;25(4):779–92.

59. Itoi T, Sofuni A, Itokawa F, et al. Peroral cholangioscopic diagnosis of biliary-tract diseases by using narrow-band imaging (with videos). Gastrointest Endosc 2007;66(4):730–6.

60. Lee YN, Moon JH, Choi HJ, et al. A newly modified access balloon catheter for direct peroral cholangioscopy by using an ultraslim upper endoscope (with videos). Gastrointest Endosc 2016;83(1):240–7.

61. Choi HJ, Moon JH, Lee YN. Advanced imaging technology in biliary tract diseases: narrow-band imaging of the bile duct. Clin Endosc 2015;48(6):498–502.

62. Larghi A, Waxman I. Endoscopic direct cholangioscopy by using an ultra-slim upper endoscope: a feasibility study. Gastrointest Endosc 2006;63(6):853–7.

63. Moon JH, Ko BM, Choi HJ, et al. Intraductal balloon-guided direct peroral chol-angioscopy with an ultraslim upper endoscope (with videos). Gastrointest Endosc 2009;70(2):297–302.

64. Choi HJ, Moon JH, Ko BM, et al. Overtube-balloon-assisted direct peroral chol-angioscopy by using an ultra-slim upper endoscope (with videos). Gastrointest Endosc 2009;69(4):935–40.

65. Tabibian JH, Visrodia KH, Levy MJ, et al. Advanced endoscopic imaging of inde-terminate biliary strictures. World J Gastrointest Endosc 2015;7(18):1268–78.

66. Slivka A, Gan I, Jamidar P, et al. Validation of the diagnostic accuracy of probe-based confocal laser endomicroscopy for the characterization of indeterminate biliary strictures: results of a prospective multicenter international study. Gastro-intest Endosc 2015;81(2):282–90.

67. Wani S, Shah RJ. Probe-based confocal laser endomicroscopy for the diagnosis of indeterminate biliary strictures. Curr Opin Gastroenterol 2013;29(3):319–23.

68. Vazquez-Sequeiros E, Baron TH, Clain JE, et al. Evaluation of indeterminate bile duct strictures by intraductal US. Gastrointest Endosc 2002;56(3):372–9.

69. Weilert F, Bhat YM, Binmoeller KF, et al. EUS-FNA is superior to ERCP-based tis-sue sampling in suspected malignant biliary obstruction: results of a prospective, single-blind, comparative study. Gastrointest Endosc 2014;80(1):97–104.

70. Eaton JE, Barr Fritcher EG, Gores GJ, et al. Biliary multifocal chromosomal polys-omy and cholangiocarcinoma in primary sclerosing cholangitis. Am J Gastroen-terol 2015;110(2):299–309.

71. Barr Fritcher EG, Kipp BR, Voss JS, et al. Primary sclerosing cholangitis patients with serial polysomy fluorescence in situ hybridization results are at increased risk of cholangiocarcinoma. Am J Gastroenterol 2011;106(11):2023–8.

72. Bangarulingam SY, Bjornsson E, Enders F, et al. Long-term outcomes of positive fluorescence in situ hybridization tests in primary sclerosing cholangitis. Hepatol-ogy 2010;51(1):174–80.

73. Baron TH, Harewood GC, Rumalla A, et al. A prospective comparison of digital image analysis and routine cytology for the identification of malignancy in biliary tract strictures. Clin Gastroenterol Hepatol 2004;2(3):214–9.

74. Voigtländer T, Lankisch TO. Endoscopic diagnosis of cholangiocarcinoma: from endoscopic retrograde cholangiography to bile proteomics. Best Pract Res Clin Gastroenterol 2015;29(2):267–75.

75. Lourdusamy V, Tharian B, Navaneethan U. Biomarkers in bile-complementing advanced endoscopic imaging in the diagnosis of indeterminate biliary stric-tures. World J Gastrointest Endosc 2015;7(4):308–17.

76. Rizvi S, Gores GJ. Pathogenesis, diagnosis, and management of cholangiocarci-noma. Gastroenterology 2013;145(6):1215–29.

77. Mukewar S, Gupta A, Baron TH, et al. Endoscopically inserted nasobiliary cath-eters for high dose-rate brachytherapy as part of neoadjuvant therapy for perihi-lar cholangiocarcinoma. Endoscopy 2015;47(10):878–83.

78. Gotthardt DN, Rudolph G, Kloters-Plachky P, et al. Endoscopic dilation of domi-nant stenoses in primary sclerosing cholangitis: outcome after long-term treat-ment. Gastrointest Endosc 2010;71:527–34.

79. Baluyut AR, Sherman S, Lehman GA, et al. Impact of endoscopic therapy on the survival of patients with primary sclerosing cholangitis. Gastrointest Endosc 2001;53:308–12.

80. Tomizawa Y, Di Giorgio J, Santos E, et al. Combined interventional radiology fol-lowed by endoscopic therapy as a single procedure for patients with failed initial endoscopic biliary access. Dig Dis Sci 2014;59(2):451–8.

81. Kahaleh M, Artifon EL, Perez-Miranda M, et al. Endoscopic ultrasonography guided biliary drainage: summary of consortium meeting, May 7th, 2011, Chicago. World J Gastroenterol 2013;19(9):1372–9.

82. Kedia P, Gaidhane M, Kahaleh M. Endoscopic guided biliary drainage: how can we achieve efficient biliary drainage? Clin Endosc 2013;46(5):543–51.

83. Perri V, Familiari P, Tringali A, et al. Plastic biliary stents for benign biliary diseases. Gastrointest Endosc Clin N Am 2011;21(3):405–33.

84. Aljiffry M, Renfrew PD, Walsh MJ, et al. Analytical review of diagnosis and treatment strategies for dominant bile duct strictures in patients with primary sclerosing cholangitis. HPB (Oxford) 2011;13(2):79–90.

85. Gluck M, Cantone NR, Brandabur JJ, et al. A twenty-year experience with endoscopic therapy for symptomatic primary sclerosing cholangitis. J Clin Gastroenterol 2008;42:1032–9.

86. Kaya M, Petersen BT, Angulo P, et al. Balloon dilation compared to stenting of dominant strictures in primary sclerosing cholangitis. Am J Gastroenterol 2001; 96(4):1059–66.

87. Ponsioen CY, Lam K, van Milligen de Wit AW, et al. Four years experience with short term stenting in primary sclerosing cholangitis. Am J Gastroenterol 1999; 94:2403–7.

88. Saxena P, Diehl DL, Kumbhari V, et al. A US Multicenter Study of safety and efficacy of fully covered self-expandable metallic stents in benign extrahepatic biliary strictures. Dig Dis Sci 2015;60(11):3442–8.

89. Irani S, Baron TH, Akbar A, et al. Endoscopic treatment of benign biliary strictures using covered self-expandable metal stents (CSEMS). Dig Dis Sci 2014;59(1): 152–60.

90. Mahajan A, Ho H, Sauer B, et al. Temporary placement of fully covered self-expandable metal stents in benign biliary strictures: midterm evaluation (with video). Gastrointest Endosc 2009;70(2):303–9.

91. Kahaleh M, Behm B, Clarke BW, et al. Temporary placement of covered self-expandable metal stents in benign biliary strictures: a new paradigm? (with video). Gastrointest Endosc 2008;67(3):446–54.

UNITED STATES POSTAL SERVICE® Statement of Ownership, Management, and Circulation (All Periodicals Publications Except Requester Publications)

1. Publication Title	2. Publication Number	3. Filing Date
GASTROINTESTINAL ENDOSCOPY CLINICS OF NORTH AMERICA	012 – 603	9/18/2016

4. Issue Frequency	5. Number of Issues Published Annually	6. Annual Subscription Price
JAN, APR, JUL, OCT	4	$335

7. Complete Mailing Address of Known Office of Publication (Not printer) (Street, city, county, state, and ZIP+4®)

ELSEVIER INC.
360 PARK AVENUE SOUTH
NEW YORK, NY 10010-1710

Contact Person
STEPHEN R. BUSHING

Telephone (Include area code)
215-239-3688

8. Complete Mailing Address of Headquarters or General Business Office of Publisher (Not printer)

ELSEVIER INC.
360 PARK AVENUE SOUTH
NEW YORK, NY 10010-1710

9. Full Names and Complete Mailing Addresses of Publisher, Editor, and Managing Editor (Do not leave blank)

Publisher (Name and complete mailing address)

ADRIANNE BRIGIDO, ELSEVIER INC.
1600 JOHN F KENNEDY BLVD. SUITE 1800
PHILADELPHIA, PA 19103-2899

Editor (Name and complete mailing address)

KERRY HOLLAND, ELSEVIER INC.
1600 JOHN F KENNEDY BLVD. SUITE 1800
PHILADELPHIA, PA 19103-2899

Managing Editor (Name and complete mailing address)

PATRICK MANLEY, ELSEVIER INC.
1600 JOHN F KENNEDY BLVD. SUITE 1800
PHILADELPHIA, PA 19103-2899

10. Owner (Do not leave blank. If the publication is owned by a corporation, give the name and address of the corporation immediately followed by the names and addresses of all stockholders owning or holding 1 percent or more of the total amount of stock. If not owned by a corporation, give the names and addresses of the individual owners. If owned by a partnership or other unincorporated firm, give its name and address as well as those of each individual owner. If the publication is published by a nonprofit organization, give its name and address.)

Full Name	Complete Mailing Address
WHOLLY OWNED SUBSIDIARY OF REED/ELSEVIER, US HOLDINGS	1600 JOHN F KENNEDY BLVD. SUITE 1800 PHILADELPHIA, PA 19103-2899

11. Known Bondholders, Mortgagees, and Other Security Holders Owning or Holding 1 Percent or More of Total Amount of Bonds, Mortgages, or Other Securities. If none, check box ► ☐ None

Full Name	Complete Mailing Address
N/A	

12. Tax Status (For completion by nonprofit organizations authorized to mail at nonprofit rates) (Check one)
The purpose, function, and nonprofit status of this organization and the exempt status for federal income tax purposes:
☐ Has Not Changed During Preceding 12 Months
☐ Has Changed During Preceding 12 Months (Publisher must submit explanation of change with this statement)

13. Publication Title	14. Issue Date for Circulation Data Below
GASTROINTESTINAL ENDOSCOPY CLINICS OF NORTH AMERICA	JULY 2016

15. Extent and Nature of Circulation		Average No. Copies Each Issue During Preceding 12 Months	No. Copies of Single Issue Published Nearest to Filing Date
a. Total Number of Copies (Net press run)		279	338
b. Paid Circulation (By Mail and Outside the Mail)	(1) Mailed Outside-County Paid Subscriptions Stated on PS Form 3541 (Include paid distribution above nominal rate, advertiser's proof copies, and exchange copies)	96	117
	(2) Mailed In-County Paid Subscriptions Stated on PS Form 3541 (Include paid distribution above nominal rate, advertiser's proof copies, and exchange copies)	0	0
	(3) Paid Distribution Outside the Mails Including Sales Through Dealers and Carriers, Street Vendors, Counter Sales, and Other Paid Distribution Outside USPS®	41	49
	(4) Paid Distribution by Other Classes of Mail Through the USPS (e.g., First-Class Mail®)	0	0
c. Total Paid Distribution (Sum of 15b (1), (2), (3), and (4)) ►		137	166
d. Free or Nominal Rate Distribution (By Mail and Outside the Mail)	(1) Free or Nominal Rate Outside-County Copies Included on PS Form 3541	34	47
	(2) Free or Nominal Rate In-County Copies Included on PS Form 3541	0	0
	(3) Free or Nominal Rate Copies Mailed at Other Classes Through the USPS (e.g., First-Class Mail)	0	0
	(4) Free or Nominal Rate Distribution Outside the Mail (Carriers or other means)	34	47
e. Total Free or Nominal Rate Distribution (Sum of 15d (1), (2), (3) and (4)) ►		34	47
f. Total Distribution (Sum of 15c and 15e) ►		171	213
g. Copies not Distributed (See Instructions to Publishers #4 (page #3)) ►		108	125
h. Total (Sum of 15f and g) ►		279	338
i. Percent Paid (15c divided by 15f times 100) ►		80%	78%

* If you are claiming electronic copies, go to line 16 on page 3. If you are not claiming electronic copies, skip to line 17 on page 3.

16. Electronic Copy Circulation	Average No. Copies Each Issue During Preceding 12 Months	No. Copies of Single Issue Published Nearest to Filing Date
a. Paid Electronic Copies ►	0	0
b. Total Paid Print Copies (Line 15c) + Paid Electronic Copies (Line 16a) ►	137	166
c. Total Print Distribution (Line 15f) + Paid Electronic Copies (Line 16a) ►	171	213
d. Percent Paid (Both Print & Electronic Copies) (16b divided by 16c × 100) ►	80%	78%

☒ I certify that 50% of all my distributed copies (electronic and print) are paid above a nominal price.

17. Publication of Statement of Ownership
☒ If the publication is a general publication, publication of this statement is required. Will be printed
in the OCTOBER 2016 issue of this publication.

☐ Publication not required.

18. Signature and Title of Editor, Publisher, Business Manager, or Owner

STEPHEN R. BUSHING - INVENTORY DISTRIBUTION CONTROL MANAGER

Date 9/18/2016

I certify that all information furnished on this form is true and complete. I understand that anyone who furnishes false or misleading information on this form or who omits material or information requested on the form may be subject to criminal sanctions (including fines and imprisonment) and/or civil sanctions (including civil penalties).

PS Form 3526, July 2014 (Page 3 of 4)

PRIVACY NOTICE: See our privacy policy on www.usps.com.

PS Form 3526, July 2014 (Page 1 of 4 (see instructions page 4)) PSN: 7530-01-000-9931   PRIVACY NOTICE: See our privacy policy on www.usps.com.

Moving?

Make sure your subscription moves with you!

To notify us of your new address, find your **Clinics Account Number** (located on your mailing label above your name), and contact customer service at:

Email: journalscustomerservice-usa@elsevier.com

800-654-2452 (subscribers in the U.S. & Canada)
314-447-8871 (subscribers outside of the U.S. & Canada)

Fax number: 314-447-8029

Elsevier Health Sciences Division
Subscription Customer Service
3251 Riverport Lane
Maryland Heights, MO 63043

*To ensure uninterrupted delivery of your subscription, please notify us at least 4 weeks in advance of move.

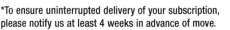
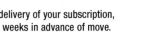

ELSEVIER